THE
FASTING PRAYER

By FRANKLIN HALL

Author of

Atomic Power With God Thru Fasting and Prayer

and

Because of Your Unbelief

NON SECTARIAN INTERDENOMINATIONAL

A MAJOR BIBLE SUBJECT HIDDEN IN PLAIN SIGHT FOR
OVER 1900 YEARS

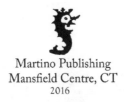

Martino Publishing
Mansfield Centre, CT
2016

Martino Publishing
P.O. Box 373,
Mansfield Centre, CT 06250 USA

ISBN   978-1-61427-958-7

© *2016 Martino Publishing*

Cover Design Tiziana Matarazzo

Printed in the United States of America On 100% Acid-Free Paper

THE
FASTING PRAYER

By FRANKLIN HALL

Author of

Atomic Power With God Thru Fasting and Prayer

and

Because of Your Unbelief

NON SECTARIAN INTERDENOMINATIONAL

A MAJOR BIBLE SUBJECT HIDDEN IN PLAIN SIGHT FOR
OVER 1900 YEARS

THE FASTING PRAYER

Order from your book seller or:

ORDER DIRECT FROM AUTHOR

Price $2.00 in U.S.A. (Elsewhere $2.25)

(Permanent address)

FRANKLIN HALL

3236 Orange Avenue,

SAN DIEGO 4, CALIFORNIA

**OTHER WORKS ON FASTING LISTED IN
BACK OF BOOK**

INTRODUCTION

"And, behold, I send the promise of my Father upon you:"

To obtain the "power," the commandment given to us by Jesus: "Tarry ye in the city of Jerusalem (your present city) until ye be endued with power from on high" (Luke 24:49) must be obeyed.

Many Christians claim the experience of Acts 2:4, but they have not attained the experience provided for in Luke 24:49. The progress so far is fine, but the deceiver still has many of us lulled to sleep, deluded, and self-satisfied, far from the goal Jesus intended for us to reach.

I once owned an airplane, but owning an airplane and getting the motor going so it will take off with its own power are two different things. If you have the Holy Spirit, He still may not have sufficient sway in your life for you to have the advanced experience of power and the gifts of the Spirit. Many do not tarry long enough, and in quite the right manner to allow the Holy Spirit to exert His power, even though He has been received. Every evidence points to the fact that the early church and apostles put into practice what the church has failed to do today. Therefore, they had an experience that overshadows ours.

After Jesus said, "I send the promise of the Father upon you" He also told them, "Tarry . . . until ye be endued with power."

Where there is a lack of perfection and refinement among God's people, as there is today, this **power** and the gifts of the Holy Spirit cannot very well be received by prayer alone. (If they can be received in this manner, I ask, where are they?) Even in the days of the apostles, they too, found it necessary at times to employ this method to arrest the flesh and become refined in order to receive this power. They were in a state of perfection that far exceeded ours today. They put into practice the prophet's-length fast and obtained the power and gifts. Without following their example and deeds, we are without their mighty experiences.

The early church-length fast acts as a refining fire to the saint of God, and enables him to become purified and cleansed to such an extent he can obtain the power and the gifts of the Spirit. It actually requires a further process of purification and sanctified living to obtain and retain the gifts of the Spirit than otherwise. The best means of reaching that goal is to do as Paul asked us to do, follow him "in fastings often." This volume endeavors to take what has generally been overlooked, reveal; and perhaps for the first time in detailed form, the secret of the early church. This is the prophet's, apostle's-length fast. It is made so simple and easy of accomplishment that anyone can have an experience as dynamic as those of any of the apostles and followers of Jesus Christ.

Joel's message predicts fasting, (Joel 2:12): "Therefore also now, saith the Lord, turn ye even to me with all your heart, and with fasting, and with weeping, and with mourning: And rend your heart, . . . " There undoubetdly will be many pillars of the faith go into fastings before Jesus returnrs, and there is every evidence this travail will bring a sweeping revival of faith, power, miracles, healings, discernment, prophecies, and other operations of the Spirit such as the world has never seen. For the day of the Lord is at hand." (Joel 1:14, 15; 2:14, 28, 29).

Enlightenment is presented upon the ten to forty day fasts. After

Jesus was baptized in water, the Holy Ghost, as a dove, sat upon Him. Up to then He had never done any miraculous thing, unless you call living without sin a miracle. Jesus still had to have something, even with the Holy Spirit, before He entered His ministry. He did not stop there as most Christians are doing today. He realized He had to have POWER. He went out into the wilderness and fasted forty days. He went on with preparation until He received power. The third day after His forty day fast, John says, He began His working of miracles. He had received power. Jesus set an example of the very thing He told us to do. It isn't enough to tarry only for the Spirit. Jesus said, **"tarry until ye be endued with power."**

When we receive the Holy Spirit, we receive only one of the two things Jesus wanted us to have.

As further proof to the fact Jesus also needed, and had received, these two important blessings in His life, we find Peter telling us in Acts 10:38: "How God anointed Jesus of Nazareth with the **Holy Ghost** and with **POWER.**"

Why should we hope to receive the Lord's better blessings and gifts of the Spirit by doing less than He did. Although the Son of God, it was necessary for Him to have a fasting experience. Have you had yours?

Brother Charles E. Robinson of the Gospel Publishing House, Springfield, Missouri, is a firm believer in the early church-length fast. In one of his letters written to me, he states: "After Jesus fasted and prayed forty days, He also received the gifts of the Spirit and went out in power and performed miracles. He did this as a man, and any person could do likewise if he followed Him all the way. Many scriptures bear this out, especially John 14:12.

"If I had a pastorate, it seems to me I would elucidate the idea in regards to the three rewards. God has a threefold foundation: Giving, Praying, and Fasting. (Mathew chapter six). These are the three things Jesus especially stresses, promising rewards. It would be a great blessing to see the assemblies practice on a greater scale the first two works, and teach the protracted consecration fasts, so Christians will fast as did the early church.

"Judging by the sermons I have heard through seventy years of listening, fasting is completely outmoded in our day. I am happy you are coming out with fasting and have a new book on same. You can't come out too strong on it. We had to do that about the Baptism in the beginning. Don't get crowded off the track it seems God has put you on.

"When I had a spell of bilious fever, and fasted fifteen days without food, Jesus completely healed my body. What I could not get done without fasting, I was able to do with fasting.

"May God bless you and this needed work."

Most deep pillars of the faith are heartily in sympathy with the protracted fast. It is the purpose of this volume to make fasting easy so anyone can go into the prophet's early church-length fast.

TABLE OF CONTENTS

ILLUSTRATIONS

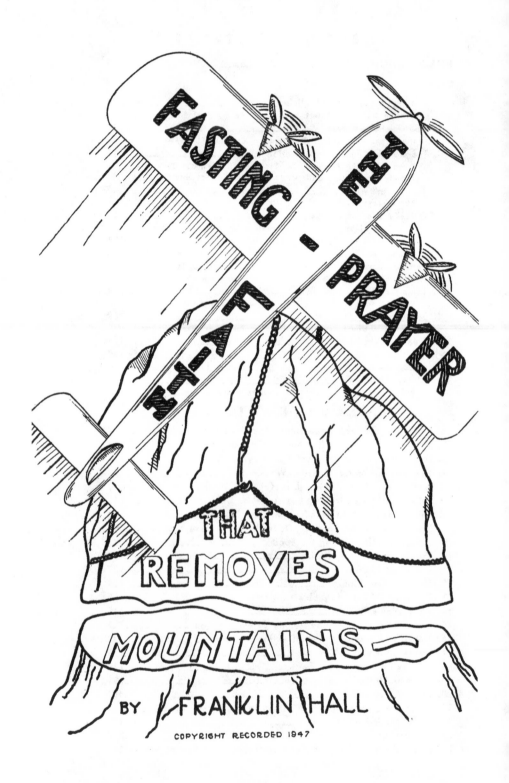

THE FASTING - PRAYER

FAITH

THAT REMOVES MOUNTAINS

BY FRANKLIN HALL

COPYRIGHT RECORDED 1947

Chapter I

FASTING MAKES WORLD HISTORY

The Lord Jehovah had certain very important plans for His people. So important were they He could not reveal them in an ordinary manner. Moses, who had been righteous and holy and had kept his flesh "under," was perhaps on more intimate terms with the Lord than any other person.

But even Moses was not capable of receiving in an ordinary manner this special package of helps and guidance that would be for the Lord's people throughout many millenniums. There was just one way by which it was possible for a holy man to approach God. He saw he could not get close enough to the Lord on a full stomach, but that He could be approached by a man completely emptied of the natural and carnal. Moses went into food abstention for forty days and was able to receive the divine commandments and instructions of God.

Later on the most God-like nations began to incorporate those same principles into their by-laws and constitutions. Today the King's Law of Great Britain are patterned almost identically according to the laws of Moses. The same is true in the Scandinavian countries. The United States has also found the precepts given to Moses to be so sound that its Constitution contains many of the same principles. In fact, most countries have many things in harmony with these great laws and commandments which were only available to a man who fasted forty days. These blessings could not otherwise have been given, because no one could have gotten close enough to God.

Every law, every ordinance, every patrolman, every officer, every judge of every nation are but symbols of what God gave a certain man because he FASTED FORTY DAYS. Every time you see a "cop," let it be remembered that he is there for your protection because one man influenced the affairs of men and nations by FASTING FORTY DAYS. Believe it or not, the lawful protection of the right and prevention of the wrong are products of FASTING AND PRAYER.

We are still under the law — not the ceremonial law, Christ fulfilled that, but we are still under the law. If a man robs another, or breaks any law of the land, we have a court that tries him, and he receives a judgment. He pays the penalty for his crime. He has to suffer the consequence. These same laws and the punishment for their infringement were patterned after the laws that were handed down from God to a man who was humble enough to approach God on an empty stomach.

Many of the greatest and most helpful blessings that enable man to get along favorably with his neighbor and fellowman are still with us. Truly this forty day fast of Moses marked a great epoch in world history for the welfare of all men and women.

A close survey of the Scriptures indicates that the deeply spiritual men who obtained great things in answer to prayer, always came to God on an empty stomach, either fasting or living abstemiously. These men made history.

Another one of God's servants who fasted forty days was Elijah. He also made history. He tried to teach the world that God was a miracle worker. He showed that none of God's saints need ever be afraid of famine if they will put the Lord first and forget about food at times. The lack of food did not bother Elijah. The Lord was so much concerned with His prophet, however, that He made a miraculous oil cruse and a meal bin to supply him with food. He sent birds from the heavens to feed him. Angels also came and prepared tables of food for HIS prophet. Although many of us have not learned Elijah's secret and his lesson, he tried to teach the world "TO GIVE NO THOUGHT FOR TOMORROW." No wonder Elijah was a miracle worker. He was in contact with God and he taught the world some very great lessons if men would just heed them.

Jesus Christ, the divine Son of God, the One whose life did more to determine the course of world history than any other, also found it necessary to fast forty days before He was fully equipped for His redemptive work.

Thousands of scholars have studied the temptations of Jesus and many comments have been made; but the fast of Jesus is never considered. His fast was inseparably connected with the temptation. This silence is neither accidental nor unintentional, for the theologians of more than nineteen centuries seem to have entered into a CONSPIRACY of silence on this very important subject. Fasting has been practiced more or less since before the time of Christ, and has been the subject of study and experiment, but nowhere do we find an explanation of Christ's fast. There exists a theological opinion, held by Roman Catholics as well as Protestants, that Jesus fasted in order to atone for our sins; but this is only a camouflaged repetition of the question, and gives no answer. If this were accepted as an answer, we would be obliged to ask: WHY did Jesus fast forty days in atoning for our sins? Did He atone more by fasting than He would have done by eating and drinking forty days?

An investigation of the history of fasting will convince one that the answer is not to be found in that direction. To whatever extent fasting has been practiced, there seldom appears any attempt to understand WHY we are to fast and WHY Jesus fasted.

An entire Jewish volume in the Talmud devoted to fasting is entitled "Taanith, Affliction." This does not contain a word that would be of any assistance in the quest for understanding of Jesus' fast or any other consecrated fast. This is composed of dry opinions of rabbis. There is no real spiritual fervor or encouragement of any kind in it. Fasts of only one to several days at the most are all that are considered.

At present the Jewish calendar lists twenty-two fast days. One of them, on the day of Atonement, is called a white fast, because each participant wears a white gown. This is a fast from sunset to sunset and is the only one that really deserves to be called a fast, because all of the other ones, called black fasts, (because black gowns are worn), last from daybreak to sunset. Food may be eaten before sunrise and after sunset. If this is fasting, one could fast all of his life by eating all he wanted before sunrise and after sunset.

Tertullian wrote a treatise on the subject in 210 A. D. In it he defends fasting as a better aid to religion than feasting. All that he urges is fine, and if put into practice would be of great benefit to the moral standard of the world today as well as to its health. He seems to consider it only as an aid in controlling the passions, however, and leaves one in the dark concerning the real spiritual power that can be obtained thereby.

Polycarp, in A. D. 110, urges fasting upon the saints as a powerful aid against temptation and fleshly lusts.

In the keeping of Lent in memory of Jesus' fast, for forty days preceding Easter, it is surprising that the Paschal fast is first mentioned by Irenaeus in his letter to Pope Victor, written in the Paschal Controversy, A.D. 195. Irenaeus states that "Some fast one, some two or more days of holy week, others forty hours (from the hour of crucifixion to Easter sunrise); this variety of observance is of long standing and existed in the time of our ancestors." Up to this date we see that fasts were mostly of a memorial nature except where used to subdue the flesh.

Athanasius, writing in the year 329, says the fast begins Monday of holy week. Eleven years later, in 340, he urges people to fast forty days as they were doing at Rome then. This was, with a few exceptions, merely abstinence from flesh food. In the year 347 Athanasius makes the statement that anyone neglecting to observe the fast can not celebrate Easter. In the fifth century we find great diversity of practice. They fasted from three to five days of Holy Week, and the weekly fasts on Wednesday and Friday were quite general.

In the sixth century fasting was no longer voluntary. The council of Orleans, 541, declared all who failed to keep the stated times of abstinence to be offenders against the law of the church. The Council of Toledo, in the seventh century, declared that those who ate meat during Lent were unworthy to partake of the resurrection.

In the eighth century fasting was considered meritorious; offenders against fasting ordinances were excommunicated; in some cases the teeth of offenders were drawn for eating flesh in lent.

The Council of Trent, 1545-1563, XXV, exhorts all to use diligence in obeying fasts, and disobedience of her commands is sin.

As an authoritive Roman Catholic verdict, St. Anthony practiced it extensively and intensively in Monasticism.

The system of fasting in the Roman Catholic Church was not founded on that of Christ and the apostles. Their

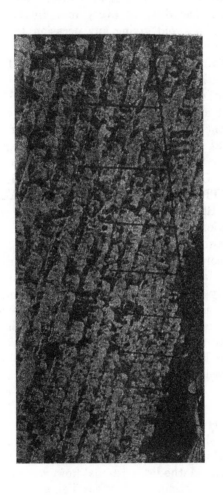

To the Mohammedans, who are a tenth of the world's population, the day of Id-ul-Fitr, on which the month-long fast of Ramadan is ended is the most sacred. In Delhi, India's capital, 250,000 believers face Mecca, Islam's Holy City, and worship in prayer to Allah, after their 30 day fast. The women standing do not pray.

millions who have fasted and still fast, do not know why
or how a Christian should fast, and so, largely fast in vain
(Matthew 6.)   We thus look elsewhere.

When we turn to the writers of the time of the Reformation we find an intelligent attitude as to fasting. The
Augsburg Confession, XXVI, states: "We moreover teach
that it is the duty of every man by fasting and other
exercises to avoid giving any occasion to sin, but not to
merit grace by such works."

Calvin, Inst. IV, 12, 14, 15, says: "Therefore let us
say something of fasting; because many, for want of knowing its usefulness, undervalue its NECESSITY, and some
reject it as almost superfluous, while, on the other hand,
where the use of it is not well understood, it easily de-
generates into superstition. Holy and legitimate fasting
is directed to these ends: for we practice it either as a
restraint ON THE FLESH, (TO PRESERVE IT FROM
LICENTIOUSNESS), OR AS A PREPARATION FOR
PRAYERS or pious meditations, or as a testimony of our
humiliation in the presence of God, when we are desirous
of confessing our guilt before Him."

According to the Westminster Confession, XXI, 5,
"Solemn fastings are in their times and seasons, to be used
in a holy and religious manner." This makes "religious
fasting" one of the duties required in the second commandment (question 109), and ordains a fast in congregations
before an ordination.

The Methodist Episcopal Church enjoins fasting or
abstinence in the General Rules, advises weekly fasts to
her clergy, and directs that "a fast be held in every society
on Friday preceding quarterly meetings." It is rarely that
anyone is found observing these rules of fasting, though
John Wesley required all ministers to promise to fast and
uphold this teaching.

Early Methodist customs, however, observed Fridays
as days of abstinence. Stevens Vol. 2, P. 134.

The Church of England has a table of fasts in its
prayer book including all Fridays, Lent, the Ember Days,
certain vigils; but merely enjoins a special measure of devo-
tion and abstinence on these days, laying down no precise
law for their observance.

It can be seen that these four Protestant Church
groups hold a more correct view of fasting than the Roman

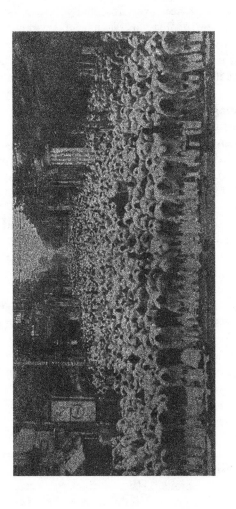

Thousands of Mohammedans offering prayers to Allah, their protector and food giver, after concluding a thirty day FAST. Ending a fast they go through the elaborate ritual of Mohammedan prayer. Such ceremonies move with almost mechanical precision because MOSLEMS pray so often and are accustomed to adjusting their movements to other worshipers. This should put to shame all saints who lack the power of God.

Church, but the practice of fasting in them today seems
too hard on the flesh and is practically nil. As the fast-
day before Communion Sunday, which was not only observed in Scotland, but in other parts of the world by the
Scotch Presbyterians, has fallen into total disuse, so also
has all other religious use of fasting advocated by the reformers, until now we can hardly find a layman, pastor,
professor, evangelist, or teacher of theology who has any
knowledge of fasting from experience. Since they do not
have this wonderful experience and do not have any idea
of what it is like, they seek to condemn it and anyone who
may have a fasting experience. They cry out against
something that they do not have, not wishing another to
put them to shame for their lack. In fact I have heard
prominent theologians declare fasting to be an unevangeli-
cal practice. The dean of a certain Northwestern Bible
College told me that it is not for us today. It was for
Old Testament times. (This was in a Full Gospel Institute).
Is it any wonder, then, that students come out of some
of our seminaries knowing less of spiritual truths than
when they entered?

Among practically all ancient peoples the abstinence
from food was regarded as a means of purifying both spirit
and body.

At the dawn of recorded history a scientific worship
known as the "wisdom religion," or the "mysteries," had
spread widely over Europe and Asia. For thousands of
years it flourished in Babylon, Judea, Egypt, Media, Greece,
Rome, Persia, Thrace and Scandinavia, and among the
Celts and the Goths.

This Religion required a long probationary period of
prayer and fasting. The Druid priests among the Celts were
required to undergo a prolonged fast in preparation for
initiation into the mysteries of their cult. In the Mithraic
or sun-worshiping region of Persia a fast of fifty days was
required. Religious fasting is practiced even today in India.
Gandhi, the great Hindu leader, has fasted frequently,
sometimes for long periods.

These earlier practices of fasting usually were associated with some form of penance and generally were part
of a religious rite. The fact was recognized that food
abstention brought men closer to the spirit realm than
any other process, as well as greatly increased vitality.

However, not all fasting of olden times was associated with religion. Avicenna, the great Arabian MOHAMMEDAN physician of the tenth and eleventh centuries, often prescribed three weeks' fasting for his patients. Especially was the fast advocated in syphilis and smallpox. At the time of the French occupation, the Arabian hospitals of Egypt were reported to be obtaining radical cures of syphilis by fasting. Dr. Robert Bartholow, although a strong believer in drug treatment, admitted that "it is certainly an eminently rational expedient to relieve the organism of a virus by a continuous and gradual process of molecular destruction and a renewal of the anatomical parts." Such is the theory of the hunger cure of syphilis, an oriental method of treating this disease. Very satisfactory results have been obtained by this means. This dreadful blood disease is being treated today by many physicians who find fasting a most important factor in the treatment of syphilis.

These Mohammedans, therefore, have a far greater knowledge of the spiritual and therapeutic value of fasting than the Western peoples. Its practice in their religion will put nearly any baptized saint to shame. If it was practiced in the churches today to the extent that it is practiced in the Orient, and among the heathen, there is every indication that the Church of Jesus Christ would be blessed with major signs, healings, and miracles all of the time, instead of just a sprinkling here and there.

The Mohammedans know how to fast. They very definitely know the value of the practice in their religion. Their GREAT PHYSICIANS have left knowledge to them that erases fear that harm could come through FASTING. How much more effectively could we, as worshipers of a REAL LIVING GLORIOUS CHRIST, utilize this FAITH PRODUCER as a means of removing obstacles from our approach to the spiritual realm.

Let us also use this medium which the Greek, Roman, and Mohammedan religions use to obtain ZEAL and FERVOR, only let us use it to glorify our most LOVABLE, FAIREST of the FAIR, JESUS CHRIST.

We are very much in need of everything that can be brought about by FASTING. Let us not be satisfied with less than the fasting "REWARD" that our "FATHER" will give us "OPENLY." We should not be any more neglectful of this opportunity of praising and honoring Jesus than any other. It surely has grieved our Redeemer that many of the children of the Bridegroom have never even fasted four days in their entire lifetime, let alone ten, twenty-one or forty days.

The Protestants should be ashamed of their neglect of this vital foundation truth of the Christian religion. The most ignorant, superstitious Mohammedans and Roman Catholics are more faithful in their practice of this sacred duty than many anti-fasting Protestant divines.

The Greek Church observes fasting with an even greater intensity than the Roman Church — the non-observance of it being the least venial of sins. The fast days here extend over almost three quarters of the year. Both the Greek Church and the Roman Church have more fervor and zeal than the average Protestant Church. This is traceable directly to fasting.

The Mohammedans have more fervor and zeal than both the Catholic and Protestant religions combined. Why? Because of the effect of the FAST. They rank higher in fasting than the combined PROTESTANT AND ROMAN RELIGIONS. Due credit must be acknowledged to them in this regard because of the place that fasting holds in their religious life. FASTING is one of the four pillars of the Mohammedan faith. During the month Ramadan, every Moslem must fast from sunrise to sunset. No food nor liquid of any kind is taken, and the time is spent in reciting the Koran or reading it. The effect of such a practice is clear to every student of psychology. Here is the reason why it is so difficult to induce them to renounce their religion. It is by this practice burned deeper into their souls through each recurring fast. This was intended by Mohammed, who was a better psychologist than many realize. He said: "Fasting is the GATE OF RELIGION." If every convert from heathenism to Christianity would spend a month in true prayer and fasting, our missionaries would have a body of such workers as they have wished for in vain, heretofore. While we give them the full truth of the Gospel, we NEGLECT THE MEANS OF PRODUCING THE FERVENCY AND ZEAL that many heathen religions have and which we do not have. THIS MEANS IS NOTHING MORE THAN FASTING AND PRAYER. ABSOLUTELY NOTHING ELSE WILL OR

CAN TAKE THEIR PLACE. IN THIS REGARD THEY ARE FAR AHEAD OF US. Shame on us!

WRONG FASTING

The zeal and fervency of the Pharisees came from the same source, — their semi-weekly fasts. Ostensibly they fasted in memory of Moses and the Law. These were also memorial fasts. In reality they occupied their minds with their traditions during their fasts, and the result was a zeal that Jesus recognized, while He was obliged to condemn severely this method of fasting. "Ye compass sea and land to make one proselyte, and when he is made, ye make him twofold more the child of hell than yourselves." Matt. 23:15. Those people were over-zealous in the wrong way. Also see Matt. 6:16:18.

A similar rebuke in regard to wrong fasting is given in Isaiah 58:3-8: "Wherefore have we fasted, say they, and thou seest not? Wherefore have we afflicted our soul, and thou takest no knowledge? Behold, in day of your fast ye find pleasure, and exact all your labours. Behold, ye fast for strife and debate, and to smite with the fist of wickedness: ye shall not fast as ye do this day, to make your voice to be heard on high." (Verses 3 and 4).

This fast was just a form, it was not a fast from the real spiritual outflow of the heart. Although zeal was manifested there was not the proper motive behind it. Their hearts were not right and it was actually a mockery to God. Their cares, toils, and labours were for selfish interests, and not for the actual GLORIFYING OF GOD. They FASTED TO BE SEEN. Jesus also condemned this method in Matthew 6:16-18. Their fasts were to draw attention to the fact that they were important religiously, and to impress their fellows that they were "somebody." Altho they "received their reward" from man, it was vain glory. (Verse 5) "Is it such a fast that I have chosen? A day for a man to afflict his soul? Is it to bow down his head as a bulrush, and to spread sackcloth and ashes under him? Wilt thou call this a fast, and an acceptable day to the Lord?" A selfish fast prompted by pride and self-interest was worse than no fast at all. God could not accept it. The poor and oppressed were suffering while the individual that was fasting for selfish motives was seeking things hypocritically from God. (Verse 6, 7) "Is not this the FAST that I have chosen? To loose the bands of wickedness, to undo the heavy burdens, and to let the oppressed go free, and that ye break every yoke? Is it not to deal thy bread to the hungry, and that thou bring the poor that are cast out to thy house? When thou seest the naked, that thou cover him; and that thou hide not thyself from thine own flesh?"

Kindly notice these fasting instructions as given here, deal with consecration and an unselfish motive. First of all, if a person would "delight in approaching to God," he must go down in humility, searching and emptying out self; he must help the oppressed and the poor; he must support the church and the missionaries; and when one's heart is truly right with God and his fellow man, he then becomes worthy to expect God to honour him with the fast. Matt. 3:8: "Bring forth therefore fruits meet for repentance," commands John the Baptist, who fasted often. (Matt. 9:14).

THE THREE REWARDS

Isa. 58:8: "Then shall thy light break forth as the morning, and thine HEALTH SHALL SPRING FORTH SPEEDILY; and thy righteousness shall go before thee; THE GLORY OF THE LORD SHALL BE THY RE-REWARD." Unspeakable glory comes after the fast. I call your attention to many testimonies to verify this point. Verse nine continues with the great FASTING REWARD: "THEN SHALT THOU CALL, AND THE LORD SHALL ANSWER; THOU SHALT CRY AND HE SHALL SAY, HERE I AM. IF thou shalt take away from the midst of thee the yoke, the putting forth of the finger, and speaking vanity," (Verse 11): "The Lord shall guide thee continually, and satisfy thy soul in drought, and make fat thy bones: and thou shalt be like a watered garden, and like a spring of water whose waters fail not." These are just some of the great rewards that can be expected as a result of the right kind of a consecration fast before God. I think they are wonderful, praise the Lamb of God forever!

These are some of the rewards that are obtained through fasting which Jesus had in mind when He delivered His sermon on the mount. Matt. 6:18: . ."Thy Father shall reward thee openly." God's people seem to want the

"REWARDS" of PRAYER and the "REWARDS" of ALMSGIVING, but they never seem concerned about the great rewards that can be had through "FASTING." Yet all three of these great subjects with which Christ dealt in Matthew chapter six, in the Sermon on the Mount, provide for rewards. These truths were high points of this sermon. Why not go after everything that God has for us?

We shall notice in detail some of the rewards of FASTing:

Spiritual "light shall break forth." A new grip on God, power in prayer, and a FERVENCY that one may never have expected will result.

"THY HEALTH SHALL SPRING FORTH SPEEDILY." Healing for the sick and afflicted is promised through fasting. What better way can Divine healing be obtained than through prayer and fasting? Matt. 17:21.

"Righteousness shall go before thee." Others will get a better glimpse of Jesus in us, and our way of Christian living will provoke others to turn to Chirst. They will see our holy life.

"The GLORY OF THE LORD SHALL BE THY REREWARD." After the fast, and many times during the fast, the joy will be unspeakable. We have a feeling of the fullness of God instead of the fullness of food. We have faith that we never had before.

"The Lord Shall Answer". Our prayers and problems have been answered, we now can shout with ease, "HALLELUJAH." "Here am I." The Lord is right beside us, ready to do more for us after the fast.

"If thou draw out thy soul to the hungry, and satisfy the afflicted soul: then shall thy light rise in obscurity, and thy darkness be as the noonday." Isa. 58:10. When the soul is bowed in humility and other conditions are met in the fast, these rewards come forth. Fasting is humbling one's self with deep consecration, and as a result the individual will be exalted. Luke 14:11: "For whosoever exalteth himself shall be abased; and he that humbleth himself shall be exalted."

There are many other rewards to be had from FASTING in the proper way, but this is not the real reason why we should fast, and is not why Jesus fasted.

Martin Luther fasted for days at a time while trans-

lating the Bible, and that is no doubt the great secret
that lies in his unrivaled translation. His great faith was
largely the revelation of God's presence which comes only
through prayer and fasting. Some of the early reformers
fasted and prayed down the old-time power, but many
people did not know this was the result of fasting. Fasting is much like faith, and few understood the scientific
side of the question. The long protracted fast like Jesus
and the Bible saints went into, was long ago lost sight of.
The Holy Word clearly indicates that the discontinuance
of the practice of fasting is in direct opposition to the example and teaching of Jesus Christ.

It was not until the first part of the last century that
fasting really became popularized, and began to be con-
ceded as something harmless and a highly valuable therapeutic measure to be applied in cases of disease as well
as a process towards reaching Atomic Power with God.

In 1822, Dr. Isaac Jennings of Oberlin, Ohio, instituted
modern therapeutic fasting. He employed fasting successfully in almost every case of disease for forty years. Many
of the early nature-cure writers pointed out the great
value of fasting in many cases of disease. Among the
chief of these were Sylvester Graham, the originator of the
"Graham floor," Dr. Fussell T. Trall, Dr. Joel Shew, Dr.
R. Walter, Dr. John Cowan, Sebastian Kneipp, Dr. Emmet
Densmore and others of the hygienic or NATURE CURE
SCHOOL. Long before this, certain physicians advocated
following the plain simple teachings of Christ in connection with temperance in eating. Tornaro, Bacon and
earlier writers emphasized the importance of a very limited
diet, and an increased number of physicians have continued
to emphasize this to the present day.

The real prominence and popularity of fasting was not
reached, however, until Dr. Edward Hooker Dewey and
a Christian Doctor, Henry S. Tanner, began popularizing
it by employing this procedure with remarkable success
in both acute and chronic disease. This pioneer work began to place an old subject in an entirely new light. It
began breaking down certain erroneous ideas of harm coming from the things that Jesus told us to do.

Dr. Tanner who was a devout Bible student, con-
tended against many medical men and theologians of his
day, that any average person could take a fast like Jesus

did. More than once he got into difficulty with both medical men and religious leaders, who seemed to stand together in denying that anyone could fast forty days and live. Dr. Tanner labored earnestly for the advancement of the cause of FASTING. To his untiring efforts and strong convictions we owe much of our present knowledge of the truth concerning fasting.

The author was privileged to meet a relative of Dr. Tanner, E. G. Phoenix, at the close of an afternoon speaking-teaching engagement on the subject of the FASTING-PRAYER in the Moore Theatre, Seattle, Washington. The auditorium along with a balcony and gallery was filled to capacity and hundreds were turned away. Fifty thousand pieces of literature were distributed as well as eight hundred copies of "ATOMIC POWER WITH GOD THRU FASTING AND PRAYER". We had a fasting prayer revival and hundred's were converted and hundreds started fasting. God healed and Baptized. Revival fires started in many other churches. (See picture of two thousand, the Moore Theatre).

Brother Phoenix told me personally after this great service:

"Thank you, Brother Hall, for referring to my uncle, Dr. Tanner, in your lecture. My uncle always believed in fasting. He put many a preacher to shame because they would not fast like the Lord wanted them to. They were always scared when he talked about fasting just for one week. One day Dr. Tanner challenged the preachers and doctors. He told them that he would prove that fasting was for us today just like it was for Elijah, Daniel, David, Jesus Christ, John the Baptist and other Bible saints. He said, 'I will prove to you and to the world, under experiment, that rather than starve to death in forty days, I shall come out of this fast in better health than when I went in.' They just ridiculed him. Anyway, Dr. Tanner, at the age of 50 and in the middle of the ninteenth century, started on his lengthy EXPERIMENTAL FAST. This was the fast that astounded the world. In Chicago, under complete observation, my uncle fasted for forty-three days without food. He certainly did shut their mouths. At the conclusion of this fast he claimed to have seen heaven, angels and the Lord Jesus Christ. Many

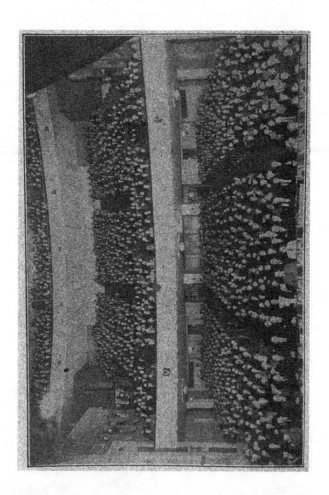

FASTING-PRAYER REVIVAL, SEATTLE, WASHINGTON, 12/29/46.
THE MOORE THEATRE. Scores of Christians started fasting ten to forty days for old time revival. Here are the results. Hundreds converted, many healed and baptized. Nearly one thousand people turned away when this photo was taken. City wide campaign by Little David and Franklin Hall FASTING evangelistic party. The author met Dr. Tanner's nephew, Brother E. G. Phoenix.

prayers were answered. He became a pioneer for the advancement of fasting. He taught it, and put it into practice with his patients. At the age of 60, Dr. Tanner fasted for fifty days. In the middle of this fast he saw the unspeakable glories of God. He came out of this feeling thirty years younger and looked only forty. Both the medical and the religious world bowed to the knowledge that he had re-discovered. At 77, Dr. Tanner took his longest fast. He fasted fifty-six days this time. Again he received wonderful spiritual revelation and glory as well as youth-restoring helps. The glories of the great beyond were accessible to him. Not many folk know this, but Dr. Tanner's thin grey hair, after this fast, was replaced by a crop of new black hair. It was the same color that it was when he was a young man. My uncle lived to attain to the ripe old age of nearly 93."

Two days before our Brother Tanner went to be with the Lord he preached his last sermon. In this farewell sermon he preached about the rewards of fasting, and stated that his longevity was due to his fasting. Thank God for Doctor Tanner who believed in putting the entire gospel to practice.

At the close of another service of the Moore Theatre and while in the process of writing this chapter during the Christmas holidays of 1946, I talked again with Brother Phoenix who lives in Seattle, Washington. He informed me that another relative of Dr. Tanner, Dr. Luzern Hinkley, of Green Springs, Ohio, has all of the original observations and experimental records of this dear Christian Doctor who pioneered in fasting, showing and proving to you and me that it is a perfectly safe and sound exercise to go into for the Glory of the Lord Jesus Christ. I personally thank God from the depth of my heart for a Christian like Dr. Tanner. Dr. Luzern Hinkley is an advocate of this truth also, and happens to be over ninety years of age. I notice that the people who fast and live the Godly life actually do live the longest.

Brother E. G. Phoenix tells me about his 40 day fast:

"Knowing so much about the fasts of Dr. Tanner and how wonderfully they helped him both spiritually and physically, I decided to go on one. I may have been foolish to make the experiment that I did, but

I started the fast in San Francisco, and decided to hike and pray all the way to Los Angeles. I started walking on the highway and turned down every car that offered me a ride. Sometimes some of the tourists who offered me a ride were very persistent, but I declined their kindness and walked every step of the way. I walked continuously. I prayed, and had a wonderful spiritual feast. I rested and at times slept while walking, strange as this might seem. God overshadowed me with His Wings of protection.

I arrived in Los Angeles before I had completed the fast, and broke the fast carefully on fruit juices, taking very small quantities at first. Before the fast I had been wearing very heavy glasses, the lenses were unusually thick. I had worn these glasses from 1905 to 1927, the year that I fasted forty days. This was twenty-one years of continuously wearing these very thick glasses. After the fast, even before the fast was broken, I could see perfectly. I needed them no longer. I had a railroad physical-examination and passed it. I secured a railroad job. I also received wonderful spiritual blessing and help, and feel better than I have felt in thirty years. Glory be to God!"

E. G. Phoenix,
Seattle, Washington

FASTING ON AZUSA STREET

Yes, the second Pentecost on AZUSA in 1906 came about just like the first Pentecost. This latter rain outpouring of the Holy Spirit started with a TEN DAY FAST AND PRAYER SEASON in much the same manner as it did upon the 120 that "continued with one accord in prayer and supplication." A few people came to Los Angeles in 1906 and started a ten-day fast and prayer season and the Holy Spirit fell. This visitor came to Los Angeles and the waves of Glory came all around. The tongues of music and Heavenly chords of harmony and counter harmony brought the sweetest music to all ears. The entire audience was just vibrating all together with this new wave of music divine. Many proclaimed it the sweetest music ever heard.

The author recently concluded a speaking engagement in the AZUSA TEMPLE, CORNER OF PALOMA AND TWENTY-SEVENTH STREETS, LOS ANGELES. Mother Cotton who is in charge, was one of the original old-time Azusa folk. This is the church to which the original Azusa folk moved from the first location on Azusa Street. Mother Cotton still has an old sign up stating: "Fast day, Friday." She fasted when the power fell forty years ago. She states, "Many of the major miracles, baptisms and manifestations of the power of God were traced directly to the much FASTING AND PRAYER."

Glen Cook, now 81, came to the author's meeting. He is another of the old-time Azusa pillars of the FAITH. He told me, "I had a room adjoining brother Seymore. I know that Brother Seymore, who was the leader of the Azusa folk, fasted for weeks at a time and only ate occasionally. There was much fasting and prayer in those days, and I believe that another Azusa could be here today if God's people would get to travailing in much prayer and fasting."

Mother Craton states, "The first thing that was done, before the power ever fell on Azusa, was a united ten day season of fasting and prayer. If there was any sectarianism, fasting broke it down."

Brother Thomas, another Azusa Street worker, states: "It had to be prayer and fasting before God came down in this wise. He heard their earnest fervent cry and then He came on the scene."

Brother A. W. Dodson of the Azusa folk tells me, "They just waited on the Lord in fastings, prayer, and the unity of the Spirit. When the Holy Spirit spoke and moved, they moved. The Holy Spirit was their leader, and when the Spirit anointed, then that person spoke. There was no demonstrational barrier; nobody shut up another or told him to sit down. The Holy Spirit was there in operation, and this was brought about through intense closeness and communion with God by everyone forgetting about food and their cares. We just drank at the Fountain of the Spirit."

A great historical development was started through fasting by AZUSA in 1906. A close study of the first and second chapters of Acts proves that there was a duplication of Pentecost 40 years ago. Obviously, when all factors are assembled and the full formula put to work, things happen. The author feels that now, today, a vast repetition of Pentecost and Azusa may be brought about if all conditions are met. The main formula to be followed will consist of fasting, next prayer, and then unity in the Spirit, in very DEEP CONSECRATION.

PRECEDENTS BROKEN, 40 YEARS AFTER AZUSA

Today, in 1946 and 1947, records have been broken in the Christian Church or in the body of Christ again. Never before in all of the history of the Christian religion have so many of God's people been seeking Him in FASTINGS and prayer. Not just a fast of a few meals, but in major fastings of ten days, two weeks, three weeks, forty days, and some have gone over eighty days. All for the glory of Christ, and to bring about an old-time revival of sinners converted, the sick healed, miracles worked and the power of God demonstrated as He wills.

In January and February, 1947, the author has spoken to fifty thousand people on the subject of fasting and prayer. One million pieces of literature have been distributed on this hidden truth, and thousands of individuals have been giving their stomachs a vacation and their bellies a holiday for the glory of God. Many have vacated the natural and moved to new spiritual heights that were never-attained before.

God has blessed our evangelistic party in the past several months, and has filled with people the largest auditoriums that could be secured. Thousands have been saved, healed, baptized and have sought God via the complete Bible route in the depth of FASTING AND PRAYER. PRAISE, HONOR AND GLORY BE TO HIM FOR EVER!

Our evangelistic party is being used by God, because we have a continuous fasting chain going on and because we are advancing this truth for the Glory of Jesus Christ.

Our entire party have fasted ten days, most of us twenty-one days. Some have gone sixteen, and some as long as forty-five days without food. I give God the praise and glory because He is giving us such a harvest of souls.

We had a great revival in Tacoma, Washington, in the Fellowship Hall seating 1800. Hundreds were turned away. One complete Gypsy family of eighteen were saved after God healed the father who is the son of the King of the

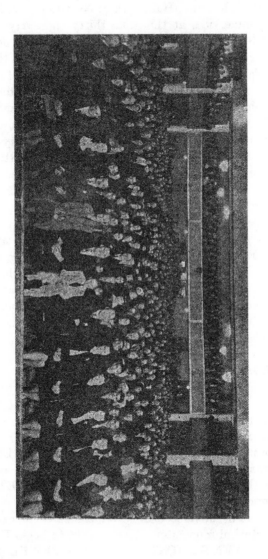

Results of FASTING AND PRAYER IN TACOMA, Wash., Feb. 2, 1947, FELLOWSHIP HALL, seating 1800. Hundreds turned away. The whole city shaken. Pastors' congregations and children began getting healed, baptized. Hundreds started fasting for a world-wide revival. One man fasted 27 days and saw all five of his unsaved sinner friends come forward and become saved. Many claim it was the greatest REVIVAL that ever came to Tacoma. Sister Mary Sommerville is here.

Gypsies, see second row in the picture. Some gypsies received the Holy Spirit.

The Little David evangelistic party have been majoring in the FASTING PRAYER. In the front row are the personnel of this party. From left to right, with hands on lap, is Franklin Hall, author. Next to myself is Sister Mary Sommerville, at this time thirty eight days along on another one of her forty day fasts. She fasted forty five days here. Next to her is Little David's father, Reverend Jack Walker, and then Little David. Next to Little David is Brother Dale Hanson, who just broke his ten-day fast for this very meeting. Later on he fasted twenty-eight days. Next to him is Sister Barbara Hanson, who concluded her fourteen day fast, and a little later a twenty-one-day fast, and had such wonderful victory in souls getting converted, she testified she never felt better in her life. Little David's sister, Mary Anne, and the three Gering sisters are at the left of Sister Hanson. They too, fasted ten, fourteen, and twenty-one days. This is why Tacoma had the greatest revival in the city's history. Major miracles, signs and wonders followed, and hundreds of sinners were converted.

We are pressing forward some things that Satan very much dislikes, and we need much prayer and fasting behind us so that we can have a world-wide crusade of FASTING AND PRAYER — real Gospel truth to march on, AMEN.

ADAM'S FAST BROKEN

One must never forget the sad plight the world is in today which was caused by the failure of Adam and Eve to continue on another kind of fast from the eating of natural CARNAL FOOD OF SIN. WORLD HISTORY was changed from the joyous communion and fellowship with God, and A SPIRITUAL LIFE ETERNAL to mortality, corruption, carnality and sin.

The adverse change on planet earth caused another historical momentous development to begin IN HEAVEN. HEAVEN'S MOST PRECIOUS JEWEL OF GLORY WAS CONCERNED. HEAVEN WAS OBLIGED TO LOSE FOR A TIME HER GEM AND CROWNED POSSESSION OF CELESTIAL BODIES. THE SUPREME BEING WAS ALSO CHANGED BY THE

GREATEST HISTORICAL TRANSACTION OF MIL-
LENNIUMS. HE WAS MUCH IN LOVE WITH HIS
NEWEST AND GREATEST CREATION, "MAN". HE,
TOO, WAS REQUIRED TO FAST FROM THE HEAV-
ENLY FOOD OF THE SPIRIT AND SURRENDER,
EMPTY, AND WITHDREW HIMSELF FROM HEAV-
ENLY GLORY; TO GIVE UP CHERUBIMS, ARCH-
ANGELS, AND HEAVENLY HOSTS. THIS EPOCH
MAKING EVENT NOT ONLY CAUSED CHANGES
IN THE HISTORY OF WORLDS, THE HISTORY OF
UNIVERSES, BUT THE HISTORY OF GOD HIM-
SELF, ALL BECAUSE A WOMAN GAVE WAY TO
THE LUST OF AN APPETITE THAT SHE COULD
NOT "KEEP UNDER."

The seed of a woman (Jesus Christ) was to bruise the
Serpent's head. Satan was enraged and from that time on
has sought to continue to work through woman's appetites
to degenerate man, nations and the world. Woman's
greatest enemy is the Serpent. She was deceived first and
led the race into death. Adam was not deceived but ate
the forbidden menu in full knowledge of the consequence.
1 Tim. 2:14: "Adam was not deceived, but the woman
being deceived was in the TRANSGRESSION."

Sin entered the race through a woman. She did not
have control of her appetite and ate the food she was not
supposed to eat. Satan is very angry with woman and
endeavors to get even with her because it is through her
seed that he is to be defeated. Another woman, Samson's
girl friend, causes the strong man of God to fall. Satan
uses the harlot Jezebel to kill off the prophets. Jesus tells
about a woman with meal (false doctrine). The first
of the Bible starts with a woman enticed by the Serpent to bring sin into the world, and the Bible ends
with another woman that is older than any other woman
on the face of the world. This abominable female also is
the WICKEDEST WOMAN THAT EVER LIVED, SHE
IS THE WEALTHIEST WOMAN, AND IS MOTHER
OF MORE HARLOTS THAN ANY OTHER WOMAN.
She is the false church. She is fully described in Revelation 17. She is the FALSE CHURCH of Christ, the mother church with her headquarters on seven hills in Rome.

She is responsible for more than fifteen million mar-
tyrs of Christ. Christians were tormented, torn in pieces,

burned and tortured in every imaginable manner during the dark ages.

Woman has more power than man to make righteous nations or cause them to fall. She can raise families into high, moral, Christ loving, righteous homes, or drag them to low standards of immorality, drunkenness, shame and infidelity. She has power to make or destroy a Godly civilization.

In the home women prepare meals for their families. It is said, "we are a product of what we eat." Wasn't this true when our fore-parents ate and caused the race to fall? Women have much power to lead families to better and more wholesome living. Their influential place in the home and kitchen is more important than generally realized. Many children and even husbands suffer, just because the lady of the house does not think seriously enough about the preparation of food that will either nourish the body or starve a person. The meal may be large in quantity, but poor in proper elements for the body. The queen of the household can be a blessing or even a curse, sometimes without realizing it.

Anyway, it is all within her power. Thus Satan is again working through women to destroy or lower the righteous standard of mankind, though many times the woman may be in ignorance as to what it is all about.

Another appetite that derives its power from FOOD, is the appetite of SEX. Food should be prepared so as not to over-stimulate the sex nature,

Again your attention is called to how Satan is using women unwittingly or knowingly, to attract the attention of the masculine sex, to pervert the mind and soul by the conspicuous showing of limbs, torso, and tight form-fitting attire. Jesus said, "Whosoever looketh on a woman to lust after her hath committed adultery with her already in his heart." Matt. 5:28. Many a female has gone down the street with an unholy, undecent exposure of some part of the body before a man. Sometimes a report in the paper comes out like this:

"UNCLAD BODY OF GIRL FOUND NEAR RIVER"

"Girl 19 Raped," etc.

Many females consciously or unconsciously entice and rouse sex lust in the opposite sex. Thousands of men who are sex perverts were made immoral through the looseness of dress, the show of form and figure, by the fair sex. They set the pace, and if men and women do not commit adultery and fornication openly, they are tempted to do so secretly through the conspicuous obscene attire of a weak-minded sister. Jesus calls this adultery. I believe the female is also just as guilty. We are living in a time of sex-daze and sex-craze,—it is also a sign of Jesus' coming in the last days. By proper eating, dressing, fasting, and living according to the plain simple teachings of Jesus, we can all go a long way toward more morality, righteousness, and holiness for His glory.

As we proceed further and deeper into this study, the reader will find it more interesting.

BLESSINGS THROUGH FASTING ELSEWHERE

FASTING IN LIMA, PERU

Dear Brother Hall,

I can say that I feel wonderful after the ten-day fast that I undertook. Thanks for the information given in your book and tracts.

Fasting worked both ways in my life. Spiritually I feel so much closer to the Lord and I feel better physically than I have felt for ten years.

Your truly,

A. S.

Lima, Peru

FROM SOUTH AFRICA

"I was so delighted to learn about fasting. Fasting is so helpful in this out-of-the-way place in obtaining many things from the Lord. The information that you have given is the first of this kind I have ever heard about. Yes, it works out just as you said that it would in the book. I would like to translate some of the tracts into the African language so that we can get the natives to understand more about it, especially the native missionaries. It will make them teachers of fasting and they can help spread this wonderful truth throughout this entire area.

A Fellow Missionary in Christ,"

South Africa.

Part of a letter from Pastor S. S. Samuel, Arapalayam
Road, MADURA G. P. O. SOUTH INDIA.

"Your tracts and book that came into my hands recently
have been a revelation to me on the consecration Bible Fasts.
I am a deep believer in fasting. You have made it possible for
me to fast much longer, to be a Daniel in power, and to have
access to Spiritual power like the other prophets and apostles had.

This is the first time that I ever heard or read anything on
this neglected subject.

This truth will be a real Spiritual blessing to all of us out
here in South India. I am going to do my part in spreading it here.

May I have permission to translate some of your material
into this language?

Please send me any other material available on this subject.
We are very much interested in it. It is truly a POWER in getting closer to the Lord. Thank you very much."

S. S. Samuel

South India.

Another letter from South America tells how the Lord
is also blessing them through fasting and prayer. Revival
fires are being kindled and saints are praying and fasting
for a great revival.

I receive letters from Canada daily of how the Lord
is blessing Bible schools, churches and various individuals
who consecrate their lives to Him in PRAYER AND
FASTING. I receive many ten, fourteen and twenty-one
day fasting testimonies of how wonderfully the Lord is
saving loved ones, healing bodies and answering prayers
through fasting and prayer.

Marvelous reports come in from all over the world
about how the Lord richly rewards His people for following
the Bible pattern of a very plain and simple truth.

Chapter II

THE FASTING PRAYER

PRAYER and *FASTING* move the hand that controls the Universe. CONSECRATED FASTING-PRAYER opens the Heart of God and the Windows of Heaven and brings the forces of God into action in your behalf.

Many of God's people are not acquainted with the most effective prayer possible. The Fasting-Prayer is far more effective than the usual prayers. The Fasting-Prayer will move God to put the Holy Spirit to work in our behalf, and will overcome apparently impossible obstacles. It is a prayer that sees your healing an accomplished fact; a prayer that is illuminating, transforming and dynamic in its results. It is a prayer that glorifies our Lord Jesus Christ and honors Him to the utmost. This is the hidden prayer, practically a lost art since the early church, hidden in plain sight for nineteen hundred years, yet it is immediately available to all of us. The most precious promises of our Lord are contingent on Prayer and Fasting.

The Fasting-Prayer leads one far beyond the realm of human conception. It transcends the natural laws and causes God to move behind the scenes with Divine Power. This prayer is so easily exercised that it can be put into practice by any man, woman, banker, merchant, clerk, laborer, servant and even a child. It is a prayer that seems like a mystery, but when we see what it is, how it works, what it does, and the accomplished results, we are amazed. Its very simplicity is what makes it seem mysterious.

It is up to you if you want to realize the benefits of the Fasting-Prayer; take a fast yourself, and pray, and watch God work.

We cannot expect more faith, talent or gifts of the Spirit until we exercise the faith, talent or gifts we already have. As we exercise the muscles of our body they develop and grow. And as we exercise our mind it develops and grows. Even so, as we exercise our spiritual faculties we will see our spirit and soul develop and grow, and our faith, talents and gifts will increase accordingly.

When we fail to exercise Prayer and Fasting we are living beneath our privileges and refuse to utilize the most potent power provided by our Lord Jesus. It is like having a check made out to you by a multi-millionaire, but it is of no value until you cash it. *The Fasting Prayer* opens a drawing account on the limitless *reserves of Heaven*. Try it yourself. Step out on *God's Promises* and see the *Holy Spirit in Operation*.

The Fasting-Prayer is the spiritual "Electric Switch" that throws the dynamos of God's great Power House into action and puts the machinery and equipment of God to work to accomplish His purpose and will.

He who fasts and prays, becomes a channel for the Holy Spirit, an instrument in the Hands of God, a yielded vessel, an anointed servant, an ambassador with His Great Commission to go into all the world . . . and to do greater things than He did.

The Prayer that we are urging upon you is the prayer that sees the "Old Man" crucified and the "New Man" resurrected, quickened, and walking in newness of life in Christ Jesus. It is a prayer that mortifies the fleshly, carnal, lustful appetites for a season so they cannot in any manner retard or impede our efforts in seeking the face of God and laying hold of His eternal promises for ourselves.

This is the *Fasting-Prayer.*

We do not underrate the value of earnest sincere prayer, — it is fine. However, one may meet with such difficulties and obstacles that ordinary prayer may not be sufficient to bring the desired victory. Therefore we should take advantage of the most effective weapon possible, for according to Christ's own words, "This kind can come forth by nothing but by prayer and fasting." Mark 9:29.

There are prayers and prayers, yet the most effective prayers are not dependent upon position, attitude, mode, manner, nor even intensity, sincerity, or fervency, all depends upon *full surrender and trust*, with complete consecration, which will subdue the natural carnal desires and make one spiritually strong. This type of prayer will be under study in this volume.

We are faced with these facts in FASTING. A complete subjugation of the flesh gets under way that seems almost unbelievable. We must keep the "OLD MAN DEAD AND OURSELVES HID WITH CHRIST IN GOD." No wonder Paul was "IN FASTINGS OFTEN." In II Corinthians 11:27, he asks us to "Be followers together of me." Phil. 3:17. "Crucify the flesh." Gal. 5:24-26; Rom. 8.

If fasting is the best method known to keep the flesh subdued, and prayer is brought forward with the fast while the flesh is under subjection, would it not stand to reason that a consecrated child of God could progress much further than when not fasting? It would be to him, THE FASTING PRAYER.

PRAYER: entreaty; a formula of worship; that part of a petition which specifies the request or desire. (By Webster).

The consecration fast, then means every thing that prayer does. One of the definitions of mortify is HUMBLE, and fasting will humiliate the flesh.

In Psalms 35:13: "I HUMBLED MY SOUL WITH FASTING; AND MY PRAYER RETURNED INTO MINE OWN BOSOM."

The FASTING PRAYER is the coordination of certain factors which, when combined, will give one THE FAITH THAT IS NECESSARY TO REMOVE MOUNTAINS, as JESUS HIMSELF tells us in Matthew, Chapter 17.

Please do not compare a three or four day fast with the protracted or complete fast with which we are dealing. One does NOT GET RID OF ALL of the fleshly appetites in only three or four days, and he has a lot of old poisonous, toxic refuse lying around in the intestines and colon that these appetites continue to feed on. The appetite lusts may have been diminished to some extent, but it usually requires a fast of at least ten days or more to give some conception of what we are talking about. A short fast of several days has its value, however to get into the FASTING PRAYER, to see the unusual miracles, signs and wonders, one should try a protracted fast and prayer season of ten to forty days.

PRAYER CHANGES THINGS. PRAYER and FASTING move the HAND that controls Heaven and

Earth. Another definition of the word PRAYER, by Cruden, is: "An offering up of our desires to God for things lawful and needful, with an HUMBLE CONFIDENCE TO OBTAIN THEM through the alone mediation of Christ, to the praise of the mercy, truth, and power of God." This definition of prayer is also related to "THE FASTING PRAYER." When a consecrated Christian goes into fasting, the FAST becomes PRAYER to him in every sense of the meaning of prayer. A thousand people could fast long or short periods, they could be saved or unsaved individuals, and not receive spiritual benefits unless they became fully yielded to God. It seldom happens, but sometimes even an unsaved individual will get so convicted that he refuses to eat. Several days may pass, and in the fast he breaks through in prayers and tears to accept God. Paul had an experience of conversion almost like this. Acts 9:6-9. Our desires are more easily given over to God in a fast than by prayer alone. Fasting is not only prayer but it is amplified prayer; it is the most intensified form of prayer. It is prayer in its deepest sense. Fasting-prayer is the real prayer team that the LORD JESUS CHRIST TELLS US WITH HIS OWN LIPS CAN PRODUCE THE FAITH TO REMOVE THE MOUNTAINS: this is mentioned in Matthew 17:19-21: "Then came the disciples to Jesus apart" (they were ashamed to ask their Master before the public) "and said, Why could not we cast him out? Jesus said unto them, BECAUSE OF YOUR UNBELIEF: for verily I say unto you, if YE HAVE *FAITH* AS A GRAIN OF MUSTARD SEED, ye shall say unto this mountain, REMOVE HENCE TO YONDER PLACE; and it shall remove; and *NOTHING SHALL BE IMPOSSIBLE UNTO YOU.* Howbeit *THIS KIND GOETH NOT OUT BUT BY PRAYER AND FASTING.*"

In other words, regardless of what the mountain, obstacle, or affliction may be, if our motive is right and prayer fails to remove it, it is because there is not enough of FAITH. What will give the faith? Jesus gives us the simple formula for PRODUCING THE FAITH, this is "PRAYER AND FASTING". In other words, that which does not respond to our wishes and desires, must respond to one who BELIEVES properly. To BELIEVE PROPERLY for the work to be accomplished, one has to go to

work to build that FAITH. Although the FAITH
BUILDER is so simple, (and this will bring the answer
to ANY UNANSWERED PRAYER that will GLORIFY
GOD AND EXALT JESUS CHRIST), many actually
overlook and pass by the formula. It is strange that the
small and seemingly unimportant little things a child
could understand are the hardest to accept. It is very
likely that our adversary, the devil is only too glad we do
not readily accept these simple truths hidden in plain sight.

Jesus Christ had FASTED FORTY DAYS AND
NIGHTS; therefore unlimited faith — the product of
the very thing that He was trying to impress upon His
disciples, was available to Him. It was this FAITH that
Jesus obtained by fasting and prayer that was powerful
enough to heal the boy. WHAT A REVELATION JESUS
GAVE TO HIS FOLLOWERS. It was not necessary in
Matthew, chapter four, to tell why He fasted, because
the time was not ready to reveal it. Here in Matthew
seventeen, Jesus opens to His disciples the GREAT
SECRETS THAT CAN BE LEARNED BY ANY CHILD
OF GOD WHO WILL JUST FOLLOW THE VERY
SIMPLE RECIPE OF NOTHING MORE THAN
"PRAYER AND FASTING." Praise and glory be to the
Lamb of God! JUST THINK OF IT, ABSOLUTELY
"NOTHING SHALL BE IMPOSSIBLE UNTO YOU . .
. . BY PRAYER AND FASTING."

The formula or recipe is so easy that most individuals
read right over it or think the word "FASTING" is
superfluous and just omit it. Even some copyists leave
this word off, thinking it is too strong for their readers or
that it was included in the manuscript by error; or maybe
it does not make any difference whether it be included or
not in the Bible. These doubting Thomases object to what
cannot be seen.

I believe Jesus knew what He was talking about when
He gave us these directions on how to obtain THE FAITH
TO REMOVE MOUNTAINS. He invites us, in Matthew
9:15, to follow Him after He left this world.

When a lady proceeds to make a cake, she will follow
the recipe right to the letter and the finished product will
be a lovely cake. She might say that since the cake is
going to be sweet, it would be foolish to use any salt in it.
By leaving the salt out, the cake would be ruined; although

the salt seemed to be a very minor ingredient.

Many of God's people reason it out in their own minds that when fasting it is difficult to pray. One gets weak, or has a coffee headache, or something else. Instead of obeying the word implicitly, and doing it, they lose out entirely on the FINISHED PRODUCT, the FAITH that would have been received if the pattern of Christ had been completely followed. Why not take the Word and digest it all, it can not hurt us. Although many sermons and books have been written concerning faith, the real FAITH PRODUCER HAS BEEN TOTALLY IGNORED IN MOST INSTANCES. FASTING AND PRAYER IS THE PROCESS BY WHICH WE MAY DEFINITELY GET THE JOB DONE.

In the *Consecration Fast* the believer gets into the spirit of fasting. Our real needs, and only those things we know God would be pleased to see us have are sought- humbly and with such confidence that we know we shall have them. The FAITH DEVELOPS, and unbelief and doubts are all cleaned out through fasting. The natural appetites subside, and as we continue the fast, determined, like Daniel, not to be defeated, we not only secure answers to our hitherto unanswered prayers, but we may receive a double reward. We may have a *vision* of *Glory*, or even see Christ as Daniel did after a three- week fast. Remember, Daniel was determined not to be defeated and kept right on mourning, praying, and fasting for twenty-one days. Although Satanic powers obstructed and delayed the answer, he knew enough not to faint and give up. Was not the reward of seeing the Lamb of God in His glorified body ahead of time a wonderful privilege? See Daniel, chapter 10.

Your attention is also called to the fact that Daniel had no selfish motives in his fast. If there is the slightest selfish motive behind the fast, one cannot realize the de- gree of success that might otherwise be expected. Daniel fasted with intercession for others; he fasted to obtain revelation concerning his people in the end time.

By having a burden for others in the FASTING PRAYER, we may more easily obtain the things that we should have for ourselves too. Giving is receiving.

By fasting we get out of the EATING HABIT for a time and learn to feast on HEAVENLY MANNA, JESUS

CHRIST. We can only acquire greater capacity for EN-
JOYMENT OF THE FOOD OF THE HOLY SPIRIT
BY GIVING UP OUR NATURAL FOOD FOR A SEA-
SON. It is possible for one to counteract the other.

A close study of this humble Prayer-Fast shows us
both go together to make it the most intensified prayer of
which man is capable.

In other words, in my study of the Word of God, I
have found a revelation of a deeper prayer to God than is
usually observed in the Scriptures concerning Prayer.

No prayer (as such), is mentioned in connection with
Jesus' experience "When He had FASTED FORTY DAYS
AND FORTY NIGHTS." However, the tremendous
power and manifestations He had at the conclusion of this
period, and the spiritual battle with Satan in the temptations from which He so victoriously and gloriously
emerged, leave us no alternative but to decide that this
great FAST WAS A PRAYER. A PRAYER IN THE
HIGHEST SENSE OF THE WORD PRAYER. A
PRAYER THAT LEFT NO STONES UNTURNED.
Jesus acquired everything He needed in this FAST. He
knew this FAST was necessary before He was capable of
beginning HIS MINISTRY.

When I speak of FASTING, please remember that
I am talking about the protracted fast, the fast in which
one leaves hunger in the background and then fasts right
on through the weakness until he gets into the fast proper
—the period in which the faster gets stronger day by day.
This is a fast of at least ten days or more. To explain
more fully: many Christians call a fast of three or four
days a long fast. They fast up to the time that hunger
is about ready to leave, and right in the middle of the weakness they experience they break the fast. Actually, at this
point, one has not even gotten started into the protracted
fast yet, and if he has a major prayer problem with God,
he has not fasted long enough to see it through. He stops
short of the victory, and fails to secure the revelations that
nearly always come with a protracted fast, as well as the
FAITH and POWER WITH GOD which may be his.
People say they fast off and on all of their life, but if they
never fast long enough to get over the weakness, and get
strong again, both physically and spiritually, they have
usually missed many blessings that they could be enjoying.

Due to ignorance and confusion on the subject, many do
not understand the better way of FASTING like they
knew in the Bible days, therefore we are minus the greater
things of God.

I shall classify the different lengths of the fast. A FAST
under twelve days is considered a short fast. A fast under
five days is very short. A FAST from fourteen days to
twenty-one days is a medium-length fast. A FAST from
twenty-one to forty days is a long fast. A FAST of forty-
five days to sixty days is a very long fast.

I have been making some personal observations and
tests in regard to FASTING for many years. It is indeed
a hidden truth, yet it is at the very finger tips of us all.
FASTING is one of the foundation pillars of the Christian
religion. It was an essential part of the very life of Christ.
The men most highly developed spiritually, on record in
the Holy Word, are those who had a great FASTING
experience with God. FASTING is mentioned in the Bible
approximately one third as often as prayer. We cannot,
therefore, go on ignoring this great fundamental.

I decided to preach and teach on the subject extensively and watch the results. Results I am certain to have.
At this writing I am pastor of the largest REVIVAL
AUDITORIUM in SAN DIEGO. I gave it a test there
for many months. I wish to state that the "WORD" that
contained FASTING was preached many times, each time
a different sermon, and it did not return unto us void. In
the first ten months of this year, we have had someone
fasting ten days or more all of the time. Many times as
many as fifty would be fasting all at once. Some would
fast two weeks, some three weeks, some twenty-eight days,
some thirty-three days, thirty-five days, forty days, forty-
two days, fifty days, sixty-two days and even up to eighty-
three days. Yes, it was amazing, and I mean they fasted
without any liquid or solid food. Only water, the pure
type of the Holy Spirit was taken, for the purpose of keeping the body clean. No food whatsoever was eaten or
drunk. I am happy to report tremendous results. In this
year we are grateful to Jesus for ONE THOUSAND SIN-
NERS who CAME forward for SALVATION. Scores received the Holy Spirit and many were healed. Yes, the
"ice" was broken on FASTING, it was broken to such an
extent that the news spread up and down the West coast.

Many a minister and critic would ask me bluntly if anyone died or got hurt. The answer was quite to the contrary. Instead of going the certain way to the grave, the people who fasted received a renewal of their strength and health. Many said, "I just began to LIVE." Those who were ill when they fasted, were healed at the end of their consecration fast. Some had as many as five physicians and were given up as hopeless with heart disorders, stomach afflictions, ulcers, tumors, nervousness, and drug addiction. They gave up their physicians and came out of the fast PERFECTLY WHOLE. Thank the Good Lord. One sister who had cancer of the liver and was given up by all the attending physicians, lay in the hospital in a dying condition. She was prayed for, after a number at the church fasted for her. Instantly the Lord healed her in answer to fasting and prayer.

A man above fifty fasted over thirty days and now looks fifteen years younger.

A sister, Maude Austin, sixty-five years of age, fasted thirty-three days and a tumor came right out of her. On the thirty-fourth day she broke the fast and now is feeling like a young girl.

Charles Allen of Escondido, fasted eighteen days and was healed of rheumatism, indigestion, and other complicated stomach disorders. After the fast he felt better than he had felt for twenty years.

These are some of the answers we gave to those who had never heard of people going on the consecration fast of twenty-one days in modern times, let alone forty days and over sixty days.

No one was hurt fasting. All were benefited, unless occasionally some person broke the fast improperly by over-eating and giving way to appetite too soon.

The wonder of it all was that in most cases the person fasting grew stronger day by day as the fast continued.

The book, "ATOMIC POWER WITH GOD THRU FASTING AND PRAYER," came off the press. The Christian proofreader who read the book started on a fast and fasted thirteen days. He stated, "I never saw a book like it." Even before it was released, orders came in for four thousand copies. Many copies were placed around the Los Angeles area, Bethesda Home of Anaheim, San Diego, and Santa Monica. Hundreds of people began to fast. This book was introduced in the Philharmonic Auditorium, Los Angeles, before approximately three thousand people and many more started fasting.

A large tent was pitched in North Hollywood, California, seating two thousand people. This was within sight of the Paramount Picture Studio. The author was invited to speak to the large audiences every evening on the subject, and hundreds received the light on Fasting.

Here is the grand testimony of nearly everyone who put this deeper praying experience to work. They proclaim it the greatest experience of their lives after salvation, and comparable only to the Baptism of the Holy Spirit. It prepares the vessel in order that the Holy Spirit may work in a bigger way. They say, "one has to experience it to know —words cannot tell how glorious it is." Now is not this just what people said about the Holy Spirit when they were Baptized a few years ago? Well we do not have it all. There is a lot more for us if we let the Holy Spirit work through a channel that is cleansed and prepared by fasting and prayer. Let us go after God's best in an earnest manner and glorify God more. Try, TASTE, and see if it is not really worth the effort. Get the rest of Luke 24:49.

FASTING IS NOT WHAT IT MAY SEEM

The general impression about FASTING is that when one gets weak, dizzy, or has a headache he is hurting himself. During the first few days of the fast, the "symptoms" seem to get worse. The individual begins to reason that eating will cure the adverse conditions he seems to be in. On the contrary, the unloading of the poisons and wastes into the blood stream (which is able to absorb them when fasting but is unable to absorb them as efficiently when eating), will be completed in a few days if the fast is continued. The average individual will continue the fast three or four days then become discouraged, give up and quit, just as this physiological process is getting started efficiently within the body. The body in most cases needs this fast very badly, otherwise the energies of the body would not be consumed by the poisons, thus causing the faster to feel weak and ill.

Spiritually speaking, it is highly detrimental to faint just when one is in the middle of the "weakness of the flesh." Paul refers to this in II Cor. 12:10: "When I am

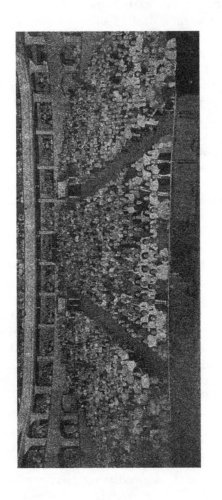

Philharmonic Auditorium, Los Angeles. A crowd of 3000 people greeted the author of the book, "Atomic Power With God Through Fasting and Prayer," when it came off the press July 5, 1946. Literally thousands of people are now fasting for a world-wide revival. The Lord's people are receiving more blessings than ever.

weak, then am I strong." Just a few verses before, Paul had
been saying, he was "IN FASTINGS OFTEN." In other
words, this very weakness that you are confronted with is
connected with the SPIRITUAL BATTLE that we all
must go through to reach the great spiritual heights that
lie ahead for those who do not faint or fall by the wayside.
Furthermore your carnal lusts of the flesh will not disappear in a short fast of only several days. These lusts
will absolutely be abolished for the time being if you fast
through this weakness of the flesh, which only lasts until
after the body becomes cleansed by the fast—usually ten
days to two weeks. (Older people require a longer time
for the weakness to disappear). In other words, there is
twenty to forty pounds of clay in the average individual
that is in more of a polluted state than the rest of the body.
When a complete fast is taken of around forty days, more
or less, true hunger will return, the tongue will become
clear, and this polluted clay will have been eliminated.
The body being thoroughly cleansed physically will at the
same time become cleansed spiritually of all doubts and unbelief, if the Christian will put forth much real spiritual
effort in prayer, with the fast. One must get into the spirit
of it and fight the good fight against spiritual darkness.
In other words, he prays through and fasts through. If
this is done one usually enjoys such victory with God that
he actually does not care whether he ever eats or not, but is
lost to the world of sense and has become abundantly alive
to the things of the spirit. Such FERVOR and ZEAL IS
engendered in worshipping God in this DEEPER FORM
OF PRAYER that there is NO ROOM FOR DOUBT
AND UNBELIEF ANY LONGER. Before the fast, we are
apt to have a lot of false ideas about "our faith," "our
spiritual strength," "our zeal for God" or our own "righteousness." The FAST will cause one really to see himself as
God sees him. We at once become conscious of our insignificance, our utter unworthiness, our weaknesses and our
insufficiency. We see ourselves in a much different light
than we ever expected. Pride, conceit, headlines, im-
patience, highmindedness, egotism, boastfulness and all
self-righteousness become as it were an ash heap after a
protracted consecration fast. See Daniel, chapter 10. II
Corinthians, chapters 11 and 12.

Certain erroneous ideas about food become fixed in a

PERSON'S mind, such as the necessity of having three full meals all the time; the stomach must always have something in it to prevent one from becoming ill; the stomach will grow together; ONE WILL GET WEAK WITHOUT FOOD AND DIE IN A VERY SHORT TIME; one will go crazy without food; we derive our strength directly from food, etc. These ideas are all wrong, and that individual who holds them is much in the need of help from God. Whether he realizes it or not, he is placing food above our LORD JESUS CHRIST. He is making CORRUPTIBLE FOOD HIS GOD.

I have personally seen scores of folk on a three-week or longer fast actually demonstrate in fact and reality that they were stronger physically than those who were saturated with three big meals a day. Believe it or not. They also became GREAT SPIRITUAL GIANTS for the glory of God. Their prayer burden for others was ANSWERED.

A lady not long ago who had not eaten a thing for fifty-eight days was so enveloped with the spiritual power of God that she leaped and shouted all over the large tabernacle for the joy of what God was doing for her in this long fast. There were hundreds of Holy Ghost filled Christians in the place who were spellbound, but this lady was super-satiated with "THE FOOD FROM ABOVE." She overshadowed them all in power and demonstration of the SPIRIT as well as physical strength.

A fast of several weeks, more or less, seems so unreasonable and such an impossible experience today, because people have never known how to fast. The average American is too busy thinking about SERVING HIS BELLY and satisfying his desire nature with *carnal,* lustful, corruptible things of the world. When the subject of FASTING is dealt with, even by emphasizing the WONDERFUL PHYSICAL YOUTH REJUVENATING EFFECTS WHICH ALWAYS COME BY FASTING, THE TRUTH IS STILL MET WITH A DEAF EAR BECAUSE IT IS TOO HARD TO BELIEVE AND IT IS NOT PLEASING TO THE NATURAL. The physical side of fasting is very *THOUGHT PROVOKING* if an individual will just look upon its scientific VALUE. The spiritual side of the subject is even MORE *THOUGHT PROVOKING* when it is studied in the light of BIBLE TEACHING AND WHAT IT HAS DONE FOR THE

MOST SPIRITUALLY POWERFUL MEN ON
RECORD. Likewise marvelous results have been obtained, and great strides have been made in our time by
those RELIGIOUS LEADERS WHO WERE NOT
ASHAMED TO DECLARE IT. Wonderful results have
followed where this portion of the Word has been honored
and practiced.

When honest-hearted people get the light on a truth it
is invariably put into practice. When I was in Hollywood,
California, I received a letter from a 'Free Methodist'
young woman who took a short fast of twelve days. It
reads: "'Know the truth and the truth will make you
free.' Praise God that His Son has set me free and
my own life can be more glorifying to JESUS
NOW.

"God had burdened my soul to FAST for my
loved ones' salvation and for my own spiritual
needs. I always wanted to fast but did not really
know what a fast was like, except a day or two.
After reading your book on 'ATOMIC POWER
WITH GOD THROUGH FASTING AND
PRAYER,' I learned some things about FAST-
ING that I never knew about. I learned how to
take a protracted FAST. I was more determined
than ever to wait upon God in fasting and prayer.

"After fasting for twelve days God revealed
Himself to me in a glorious way such as I had
never witnessed before. I was praying in the
Spirit when *Jesus appeared to me.* I saw the cross
to my right and JESUS PLEADING WITH THE
SAINTS TO GO TO THE RIPENED HARVEST
FIELDS, WHICH APPEARED BEFORE ME
IN EVERY DIRECTION. An agonizing burden
came upon me as I realized innumerable multitudes of people were dying without Christ because
the saints no longer had a burden for the lost. The
Scripture tells us, 'The fields are white unto harvest but the laborers are few.' This Scripture came
upon me so forcibly. I tried to touch Christ en-
treating Him to send laborers, but my arms were
paralyzed and would not move. The saints told
me I was prophesying in the Spirit.

"Hunger left me after the third day, the habit

hunger left me a few days later. On the tenth day of my fast, weakness left me.

"This fast was one of the biggest experiences of my life. I entreat all who read this testimony to FAST AND PRAY AS NEVER BEFORE THAT GOD WILL SEND LABORERS INTO HIS HARVEST, for truly the harvest is great but the laborers are few."

Miss Thelma Bowen,
Anaheim, Calif.

GIVE YOUR STOMACH A VACATION

When does your poor old stomach ever get its rest? It is perhaps long overdue and the need is very great. Many folk talk about taking a vacation or having a rest, but strange as it may seem, although they may travel several thousand miles or take a voyage, they actually come back from the trip more tired and worn out than they were before they started.

It is the purpose of this volume to show the reader how a real vacation can be taken, a vacation that will be as different from the ones he may be accustomed to as the day is different from night. It will be a holiday that can be appreciated afterwards, more than tongue can tell or words can express. It will be a vacation for the organ that is MADE TO WORK HARDER THAN ANY OTHER IN THE ENTIRE BODY—the stomach. This organ is made to slave for man almost night and day. Even before we go to sleep, it is usually put to work with a mess of food thrown into the food cavity, the mouth, and on down into thirty feet of tubing. Often it is busy in turmoil and unrest all through the night and when it is just about ready to relax, the morning comes and into it goes what is generally called a "BREAK FAST." To the stomach, however, it is just another conglomerate mixture. It is received into the stomach and accepted in about the same way that a hog receives his garbage. It seldom, if ever, has an opportunity to get its rest. Sometimes an individual lives a whole lifetime and his poor old belly has never received a decent rest. I am talking about a vacation of ten days, two weeks, three weeks or even forty days.

Give your stomach a vacation and VACATE FROM THE NATURAL TO THE SPIRITUAL. This would certainly be a quicker method of obtaining the heavenly riches from God than any other, because you are absolutely surrendering every bit of carnality, pride and the weaknesses of the flesh which are enmity against God. This would be a vacation supreme, with the power of God within reach of the candidate. A holiday such as one never dreamed possible would be at the individual's command. This would be utopia to the physical body and all of its organs, but to the child of God in consecration, it would be another type of prayer and spiritual power unbelievable.

Declare a STRIKE against eating for at least a week or more, and better still, go two weeks or more. Go into a hunger strike for the glory of God and strike out the devil and his powers for the time being, so that new avenues will be opened up toward heaven, and God can display His power to us in the biggest manner possible. Go into FOOD ABSTENTION and be prepared to enjoy the Heavenly Manna to the limit of your capacity.

Give your stomach a vacation. Permit it to consume all excess food poisons and to eradicate all of the many other foreign substances within that sickness and disease breed on. Old particles of tainted food lie around in the body for many weeks and cannot be eliminated because of the work and labor of taking on more food so frequently. In other words, give your stomach a vacation and let the temple of the Holy Spirit undergo a HOUSE CLEANING.

When the stomach is given a vacation from the natural, carnal things, a spiritual HOUSECLEANING GETS under way so that the works of the flesh are mortified, and unbelief and doubt are cleaned out. The child of God can then approach by every avenue possible the more blessed things of the Spirit. It may be divine healing for the body that is desired. Whatever it is, Jesus will be on the scene to meet that need.

By giving your stomach this kind of vacation you go into fasting. To the Christian who is seeking more of God, it is THE FASTING PRAYER.

It never was intended for man to be continually, all of the time, on a three or four meal a day stuffing program. The more we stuff, the more of faith and things of God we stuff out of our lives, and the easier it is to falter and faint when it comes to the things of God and spiritual progress.

Food abstention permits prayer to operate at its capacity and guarantees PRAYER EFFICIENCY TO ITS MAXIMUM.

"MEN OUGHT ALWAYS TO PRAY, AND NOT TO FAINT." Luke 18:1. A person goes to praying for something which he knows is in accordance with the will of God. Perhaps it is for bodily healing or for some other need. He prays earnestly and the prayer is not answered. He discontinues praying so earnestly about it, or he may quit praying altogether, yet he knows it is the will of God to answer. If it is in regard to a bodily affliction, it is very definitely pointed out that it is the will of God to heal the condition, regardless of how impossible it may seem in the natural, because of God's Justice, Mercy and Righteousness. If Jesus healed folk in His time and would not heal us today, He would be a respecter of persons; this would show partiality. Jesus Christ obligates Himself to heal us now just as He did when He walked the shores of Galilee. He cannot be partial. He would be an unjust God if He did not heal bodies today. Is He unjust? Of course He is not. So let us have fixed once and for all in our minds that it is His will to heal and answer the prayers that we know are in accordance with His plan and purpose.

When you pray for healing and healing does not come, it should stimulate you to seek Him harder, rather than give up and "FAINT." "Shall not God avenge His own elect, which cry day and night unto Him, though *He bear long with them?*" This is important, and fasting carries it through. There is not the slightest reason to slack down on the prayer but there is every reason to press on even into deeper and more earnest praying. The word those who "CRY DAY AND NIGHT UNTO HIM ARE AVENGED." This means that it will be necessary to get into such a spirit of prayer that FOOD AND EVERYTHING ELSE IS FORGOTTEN BUT GOD. It cannot mean anything else but a FASTING PRAYER, and THIS WILL ABSOLUTELY GET THE RESULTS WHEN ORDINARY PRAYER FAILS.

When the Lord sees this kind of prayer in action, as is sometimes necessary, ("This kind can come forth by

nothing, but by prayer and FASTING." Mark 9:29), then
God shall avenge His own elect. Luke 18:7. "I tell you
that He will avenge them speedily." Luke 18:8. It is absolutely necessary that God honor His own word and it
has to be answered. There cannot be the faintest particle
of a shadow of doubt that it will be answered. It must—
MUST BE ANSWERED. Your healing is actually on
the way the moment you realize it must be done. You
cannot be defeated, so continue pressing harder and harder
at the objective in the FASTING PRAYER. If you
should faint or let down even a little bit it will mean more
defeat the next time you have a prayer problem, and it
will mean actually less faith than you had before the start.

Our CHRISTIAN EXPERIENCE IS A "GO
AHEAD" PROGRESSIVE on-the-run BATTLE ALL
THE WAY THROUGH. We cannot give up or let down
in the slightest manner. On the other hand, when we do
press on and continue praying day and night if necessary,
and then on into a major FASTING PRAYER experience,
the victory of FAITH OVER SATAN AND THE
POWERS OF THE DEVIL WILL BE SO GREAT that
we will be amazed at seeing the victory accomplished and
our healing realized. We will obtain such power and become such WARRIORS that the next obstacle will seem
small and will easily be overcome. One victory leads to
other victories, and makes each successive conflict more
easily won. We only need to win the one or two seemingly
impossible battles and the FIGHT IS OVER, so to speak,
because all future SPIRITUAL FIGHTS seem small. The
first battle is the hardest. The fight ends in a glorious victory and is the means of many future victories. WHY?
Because the old devil has been licked. But it may require
the deep FASTING PRAYER, which so many of God's
children know so little about. However, many are trying
out this beautiful last day experience.

Again to Luke 18:8: "NEVERTHELESS WHEN
THE SON OF MAN COMETH, SHALL HE FIND
FAITH ON THE EARTH?" If there will not be "FAITH
ON THE EARTH when the SON OF MAN COMETH,"
there must be some reason why there will not be? Yes, just
a few verses back in Dr. Luke's same book, we notice the
reason why? Chapter 17, verses 27 and 28: *"THEY DID
EAT*, THEY DRANK, until the day that Noe en-

tered into the ark, and the flood came and destroyed them all. Likewise also as it was in the days of Lot; *they DID EAT*, they drank, they bought, they sold, they planted, they builded; But the same day that Lot went out of Sodom it rained fire and brimstone from heaven, and destroyed them all." The key to the entire corruptible set-up that caused the destruction was their APPETITES. Few there be that can see this because too few have ever fasted long enough to know what it is all about. If a vote were taken in the average church and the question asked, "How many have ever fasted ten days without eating any food whatsoever (water only taken)?" the answer would very likely be "NO ONE." Yet the one hundred-twenty fasted many days in the upper room. Please search the Scriptures and try it out so you can know. In a ten-day fast the appetites will have disappeared so that all of the other things mentioned in the above scripture will have no hold upon the candidate. He will not be interested in "building," "mixing drinks," "buying," "selling," "planting," "marrying wives," and of course he will not be eating because he will be in a "FASTING PRAYER" and will find such a treasure house of joy that what has been mentioned will honestly seem like "rubbish" compared to the GLORIES AND REVELATIONS OF THE GREAT BEYOND.

Here is the testimony of a very precious sister who attends the Auditorium of which I am pastor, and I know she fasts often and is mightily used of God in healing and in the exercising of other gifts of the Spirit.

"I praise Jesus for giving me the light on the FASTING PRAYER truth. The Lord was so real to me on my last fourteen day fast. He was so close and precious. I have been blessed in such a manner that it seemed HEAVEN just opened right up in my lap. Wonderful revelations have come to me and I am realizing my prayers answered. It is so real when we worship Jesus in a fast that words can not describe it. One should try it out and see for himself.

Sister Marie Gray,"

San Diego, California

Ordinary prayer becomes amplified many times

through FASTING. The fast in itself is prayer to the devout Christian. Fasting in the Scriptures is so closely related to prayer that it is taken for granted as prayer. Matthew 4:2: "And when He had fasted forty days and forty nights, He was afterward an hungred." There is no mention that Jesus prayed when He fasted, but we are certain that He did and that this fast was PRAYER to Him — PRAYER in the highest sense of the word. Fasting intensifies the POWER OF PRAYER. In Acts. 1:14: "These all continued with one accord in PRAYER AND SUPPLICATION." They were fasting also, and this made it the "greater prayer" that was followed with the dynamic "RUSHING MIGHTY WIND EXPERIENCE." They had a "SUDDEN;" a "FILLED;" a "FIRE" experience. In Acts 10:2 It is said of Cornelius: "A devout man, and one that feared God with all his house which gave much alms to the people, and *prayed to God alway*. He saw in a vision evidently about the ninth hour (3:00 P.M.) of the day an angel of God coming in to him, and saying unto him, Cornelius. And when he looked on him, he was afraid and said, What is it, Lord? And he said unto him, *Thy Prayers and alms* are come up for a memorial before God." THE FASTING PRAYER had been in action here, although it was not named. For more proof that Cornelius had been in a fast and that fact can be verified as such, please read Acts 10:30: "And Cornelius said, Four days ago I was FASTING until this hour; and at the ninth hour I prayed in my house, and, behold, a man stood before me in bright clothing, And said, Cornelius, THY PRAYER IS HEARD, and thine ALMS are had in remembrance in the sight of God."

Peter had been in a fast, evidently, because "Peter went up upon the housetop to pray about the sixth hour; (noon) And he became very hungry, and would have eaten; but while they made ready, he fell into a trance, AND SAW HEAVEN OPENED." Acts 10:9, 10. Here is another instance of a FASTING PRAYER because people who are eating regularly do not become "VERY HUNGRY." If this had not been unusual in Peter's case I do not believe the Scriptures here would have given it such recognition. Furthermore, visions or trances usually are only received when one is emptied sufficiently of the natural and carnal elements of the world to be in a receptive attitude to receive the SPIRITUAL things of God. The best way to do this is in a fast.

I have seen hundreds of people fast, not just three or four days, however some great results are received from these, but I have seen them fast many days and weeks, and in nearly all cases great revelations are received from God. In addition many have visions and trances.

If one gets that close to God, His OWN words of revelation and prophecy may be heard. Even certain hidden mysteries are revealed. The word of God becomes quickened and misunderstandings are cleared up. (Romans 16:17, 18). Furthermore, many new revelations come directly from God which are not contrary to the Bible but always in harmony with the Scriptures. These new revelations are also the word of God because they come from Him. A prophetical forecast of future events often is received by very deeply spiritual saints. Many men in olden days became prophets through fasting. Why can not we also be chosen vessels by FASTING?

I have also been surprised to see people that fasted several weeks, who were not as spiritually highly developed as might be expected, come out of a fast receiving many revelations. A person spending five or six hours a day or more in real prayer, with a fast, can receive much more from the Lord than one who prays only moderately.

I visited a spiritual sister who had been fasting sixty-four days. She had been in the process of breaking her fast with grapefruit juice diluted with water, and part of the time she was using oatmeal gruel. She told me that her experience was so gloriously thrilling in the Spirit that she even hated to break her fast. This was about a week afterwards. Two weeks later I called on her and she was in such a sweet spirit. She told me that for three and one-half hours the Lord was giving her deep revelations, one right after another and many were prophetic. Before she broke the fast she had many revelations of the great glories beyond. "It seems like I have been in heaven ever since I fasted above the thirty-ninth day. Every day since then has been too glorious for words."

The joy and ecstacy of the great victory that was accomplished on this lady's fast almost made her dread to break her sixty-four day fast. She felt that when she would break her fast she would lose all of this unusual

super refilling of the Holy Spirit and power as well as joy.
When she first received the Baptism of the Holy Spirit
it was very wonderful, but she had not gone into the
FASTING EXPERIENCE WITH THE HOLY SPIRIT.
Her experience at this time was far greater than at the
time of her Baptism, because she was with the Spirit in
His fullness and power. She was pressing along into the
deepest of experiences. A MAJOR FASTING PRAYER
that topped all experiences with God, except of course
actual translation. Hundreds of people who watched her
from time to time almost envied her and thought she was
about to become translated because the Glory of the Lord
was shining on her so remarkably.

When the lady did break the fast however, she was
so delighted to know that a great deal of the precious manifestation was retained and much of the power that was
given to her. She said, "I can pray for folk away from me
and receive answers to those prayers more easily now than
I could formerly do by laying hands on those that were
near me before fasting."* Thus the power of prayer became
illuminated in her life to the maximum.

Fasting puts legs to our prayers and gets results that
are as powerful as "ATOMIC ENERGY." Fasting ener-
gizes prayer to such an extent that the FAITH is produced that will remove the mountains, the hindrances, the
complications, the doubts and whatever else that may be
obstructing our passage way to GOD.

The FASTING PRAYER is importunity and is the
"key" given to us that guarantees, absolutely, the job will
be done when all other means fail.

As the dry parched ground needs the heavenly showers
of rain, so does the Christian need the FASTING experience to assure himself of the Faith and the great
blessed showers of the Holy Spirit and power and to keep
filled in a super way with the Spirit. As the day needs the

---

*This is the same lady who (while fasting forty-eight
days) anointed and dedicated the Author's book. "Atomic
Power with God Thru Fasting and Prayer." She obtained
a vision and a revelation of the blessings the book would
bring to others everywhere.

sunshine to light it up with cheer and happiness, so does the child of God need the FAST to illuminate him with more of Heaven's Glory, more of zeal and fervor, and more of the FIRES OF THE HOLY GHOST.

I am well aware of the fact that many of God's people as well as certain ministers argue that there were really only a few Bible characters who ever knew much about the fast, and that the author is placing too much stress on the subject. These people do not know very much about fasting and the value of the power there is in the Word of God concerning the truth when properly applied. They are much in need of fasting. This "HUSH" about fasting explains why their church is so powerless. A vital truth as important as fasting cannot remain indefinitely in the dark when a few of God's children have tasted and seen what it will do. The same thing happened when the Baptism of the Holy Spirit fell on Azusa Street in Los Angeles forty years ago. Certain ones wanted a "hush hush" concerning Him and they thought it might be alright for a few deep folk to obtain, but did not want too much publicity about HIM among all Christians.

CONQUER THE FLESH OR THE FLESH CONQUERS YOU

Those who would condemn the importance of major FASTING are not aware of the great power there is in it to whip the flesh into line. Our flesh has to be subdued and mastered and kept in line continually, or the first thing we know, we are gradually losing ground in the spiritual.

The old man is really a problem; he fights back and is very persistent in rising up to show us what a big guy he is. FASTING is the effective process that will get him under, and make him very weak. FASTING is the best means known to keep us sanctified. By FASTING a child of God can keep consecrated and more consecrated to the Lord. FASTING becomes self-chastisement to the believer. It will many times prevent God from chastising us in His way. Much has been said and written about chastising, consecration, sanctification, and many other works, graces, and fruits, but when a careful analysis is made, FASTING and prayer will go further than all other means combined to develop and complete these virtues.

Yet this most powerful of all methods is placed farther into the background and there is less written and said about it than any other subject in the Scriptures. The reason is evident. Too many of these writers and speakers, and many are excellent in that line of work, have never gone into a fast of ten days or more to taste of these beautiful experiences for themselves.

While awaking in my hotel room this morning in Spokane, Washington, where I am on a speaking tour in six large school auditoriums in and around this area, an exposure of carnality came to me that I shall use in a chart. I call it "The Food Babies." Please refer to it at this time. It may assist in revealing how powerful a place food has in our lives. It shows the appetites in a different light. The appetite of.hunger is of course the most powerful of the appetites. It feeds all the others. Food is the key to all of the appetites. Please note that the craving of our spiritual nature is almost smothered and crowded out by the abnormal physical appetites. In fact there is a separation noticed by the source of supply extending from the power of God to the soul and spirit.

If God's people would only fast ten days or more, every now and then, there would not be the backsliding, the powerless conditions, and the lukewarmness that is increasing among His people.

This chart reevals a shocking condition. It was not made as strong as Paul did in Philippians, chapter three, "have no confidence in the flesh," (3:19) "Whose end is destruction, whose God is their belly, and whose glory is in their shame, who mind earthly things."

It actually is impossible to understand all of Paul's writing unless one goes into at least one major fast. You may think you understand them, but fast at least ten to twenty-one days and see if you do not receive a different light on many of his sayings.

Our body becomes more pliable toward the Spirit and is more closely related, is more flexible and adaptable to the Spirit while on a fast than at any other time.

A colored sister had a battle with the flesh on a sixteen-day fast. She stated: "I fasted many times but this last fast brought me up against things of the flesh concerning pride and selfishness more than any other. I went on a hunger and a thirst strike (11 Cor. 11:27) for ten days and then continued the fast for six more days with water. All of the pride was taken out completely. The testings were severe, but I would take nothing for the experience that I realized on this sixteen-day fast. I can preach better and have more anointing than ever and have God in my life in the most precious manner. I also was healed of cancer."

Sister Williams

San Diego, California

Religion, more than any other existing institution in the world today, is challenged by the new atomic age. For atomic energy is the ultimate physical force, and religion is, or should be, the controlling spiritual power over all physical things. Should that spiritual power fail to control the physical forces of destruction, then this world is doomed.

THE HOPE OF THE FUTURE DEMANDS A SPIRITUAL AWAKENING, a spiritual rebirth of individuals — not any more of the unsaved than of the ones who bear Christ's name. It will require more than just an ordinary praying experience. If it comes about it will take a major praying experience — the FASTING PRAYER. There must be a revival of the Spirit.

Statesmen labor hard and unsuccessfully to remake a devastated world. Scientists and military men, more than the preachers, prove that a revival of the Spirit is necessary if the FLESH IS TO BE SAVED FROM TOTAL DESTRUCTION. The way to do this most successfully is to keep the flesh subdued, surrendered and fully mastered. Failure in this line will mean the destruction of both flesh and spirit. Or in other words, the flesh will master us.

We have already shown that the most successful manner of keeping the flesh submissive to the Holy Spirit is by FASTING.

We lost heavily in World War I when we surrendered liberties which were never regained. We lost very heavily in World War II when from us were taken priceless heritages of freedom, many of which never will be restored.

Free enterprise? Look at what has happened to American life. OPA limits the prices we may charge for meat and automobiles. OPA limits or denies profits in business.

We are told what we may charge, and what we may pay for the apartment or house we rent. If we want to build a house we must get a permit, which stems all the devious way from Washington.

Americans have abhorred the concentration camps, yet we had them right here where thousands of American citizens who happened to have Japanese ancestors were incarcerated. We had these camps for conscientious objectors. No doubt another war would see an extension of these devices.

The United States Army Air Forces, working in hand with civilian manufacturers, are developing experimental aircraft designed to explore the field of hypersonic speeds.

For example, there is the XSL, planned to double the 760 miles-an-hour speed of SOUND. This is but the first step. Other supersonic planes are being developed for even greater speeds. Already, men of the Air Forces are thinking about speeds up to four thousand miles an hour.

Why are we so concerned about speed? Because speed has become a valuable servant of mankind. Speed brings distant places close together. Speed hastens progress by eliminating wasteful time factors. Most of all speed is supposed to mean protection for the nation.

Everybody's heart is filled with fear for looking after the things that are coming upon the earth.

There is a very efficient method found in the Scriptures to step up the spiritual progress of man to equal his physical inventions and the strides of natural progress. This something is the focusing of our spiritual natures on Jesus Christ through FASTING AND PRAYER, and getting our flesh in tune with the Spirit.

Since man's natural development is so far ahead of the spiritual, it is more imperative than ever that he go to FASTING. I say that it is more important to FAST today than it was in the time of Christ. It is the only way that can bring about a quick national revival that is very necessary before the Russian Bear forces itself upon us.

America is badly drunk with "FOOD INTOXICATION." People are literally super saturated with the three and four meals a day stuffing habit. What little faith many a Christian has left, will be stuffed out with food. So saturated with food poisons and toxins are the American people that intense praying to God without fasting is an almost too difficult task to do any more. With many of the preachers it is even worse. There is seldom any denunciation of sin in the pulpit any more, but there are plenty of chicken and turkey dinners.

The hunger lust is so prevalent everywhere that there is seldom a cry against it. Approximately seventy-five percent of the individuals that comprise the line for divine healing are not healed, because, if they were healed they would go out and stuff themselves sick again. They would place in reverse in a few weeks what God had done for them. "All his days also he eateth in darkness, and he hath *much* sorrow and wrath with his sickness." Ecc. 5:17. These seventy-five percent of afflicted people need reformation as well as prayer for their healings. They need to go out and do what Jesus told them to do, FAST. (Matt. 9:15). Fasting is the greatest natural curative agent known to man and will cure most of the functional ailments people have without the necessity of going to God in prayer about it. I personally feel it is very displeasing to Jesus Christ for ministers and workers to continually pray and pray for people over and over many times when their case could be disposed of by a FASTING PRAYER. James chapter 5 includes this: "Is any among you afflicted? Let HIM PRAY." (Also Matthew 17:20). If one is sick and is able to pray, he should pray. If the job is not done he should FAST AND PRAY. Any one that is too lazy to pray and fast himself needs no healing and those who know how to pray need not pray for his healing, but should ask God to have mercy on his lazy soul. There are, however, exceptional cases where this would not apply.

The people of America are so overfed at the present time that the average person would have to FAST more than forty days, if he took a complete fast — a fast that would last until hunger would return. It might take fifty or sixty days or even longer, because the more filth and poison one has in his body, the more weight he has, the longer it requires for hunger to return. In Christ's time the average individual would have found that his hunger would return in approximately forty days of fasting. People had more muscular development. They worked harder and were in better physical trim than people are nowadays. We are in the machine age that began with the dawn of the aquarian age which we are now entering. This began to manifest itself around 1848 A.D. It will even be some time yet before we come into it fully. The machine does the work for us now, while in Christ's time man depended more on the beasts of burden and upon his own physical strength to get a job done. Consequently, today man does not need "FOOD FUEL" to the same extent that he formerly did. *This fact should more than ever induce men and women everywhere to fast more often and live more simply* insofar as the consumption of food is concerned. "All the *labour* of man is for HIS MOUTH, and yet the appetite (soul) is not filled." Ecc. 6:7.

Let us adapt ourselves to the age that we are living in. Above everything else we should realize more than ever that we are living in the closing days of the HOLY SPIRIT DISPENSATION. The time is at hand when JESUS will soon be coming upon the scene. Yes all real fired-up Christians have a shaft of hope. Soon something will suddenly appear out of the sombre skies above. With great joy and gladness will the dead in Christ spring forth, and we that are alive will be changed and will be caught up to meet the most precious GEM of our heart, JESUS CHRIST our SAVIOUR AND REDEEMER.

Yes, if Christian men and women ever needed to pray and fast and to prepare themselves for the Bridegroom, it is now. It is easy to see that within the present age it should be easier to fast than in Christ's time. The majority of us require less fuel. We have more leisure, less hard physical work to do than formerly. Shall we get into the swing of it and have more staunch men like Elijah, Daniel, David, and Paul who were "IN FASTINGS OFTEN."

For Christian men and women it should be the message of the hour.

John the Baptist, the forerunner of Jesus at His first coming, was the one who, blazed the trail and heralded with advertising the great coming of Christ. John was the great messenger who "Prepared the way" before Christ. "The voice of one crying in the wilderness, Prepare ye the way of the Lord, make HIS PATHS STRAIGHT." John did baptize in the wilderness, and preach the bap-

tism of repentance for the remission of sins." Mark 1:2, 3.
"And John was clothed with CAMEL'S HAIR, AND
WITH A GIRDLE OF SKIN ABOUT HIS LOINS: AND
HE DID EAT LOCUSTS AND WILD HONEY." Mark
1:6.

John the Baptist had a two-purpose message. This
was repentance for the unsaved, and the preparation of
God's people for the Kingdom of Heaven. The message
to the man of God was to walk straight and "PREPARE
YE THE WAY FOR THE LORD." Mark 1:3. The message of the hour, then was seeking the Lord in prayer and
fastings. Go the limit in becoming fully prepared for His
coming. Let nothing be undone that would make a person
more upright and holy. Search yourselves, forsake the
crooked paths of the world and straighten out the paths
of righteousness. Whatever there was that could make a
person more righteous, more holy, more upright, more
meek, more humble, more prideless, more loving and God-
like, these were what John the Baptist preached to the
righteous. FASTING WAS A METHOD TOWARD
REACHING THIS GOAL AND WAS MOST SURELY
EMPHASIZED AS WELL AS the proper simple manner
of life. John was so devout and earnest in his simple, plain,
unadulterated teaching of the truth that he practiced it
himself; his disciples and followers also put it into practice. John dressed simply, he ate simply, when he did eat.
His two-course meals constituted a very simple menu.
Most of the time it was "locusts and wild honey."

John's disciples were also acquainted with the power
that FASTING BROUGHT. In Matt. 9:14: we read,
"Then came to Him the disciples of John, saying. Why
do we and the Pharisees FAST OFT, but thy disciples
fast not?" The answer that Jesus gave was only an encouragement for us to fast when the Bridegroom is gone.
Surely just before He returns there should be a re-em-
phasis of fasting and prayer. The message that the wonderful fore-runner of Christ preached was the message of
preparation. If God's people ever needed to pray and fast
it is today, just before Jesus comes. Every one's heart
should literally burn with zeal and fervor to such an extent that there would be a shaking up of the church. There
should be an honest-to-goodness revival among the Christians so that "PRAYERS DAY AND NIGHT" AS WELL

AS FASTINGS, WILL CARRY up their sweet aroma to Jesus until He will feel obligated to return for His precious ones who are waiting and yearning for the SOUND THAT SHALL shake the heavens. This will be a sound of joy to everyone ready and filled up with the "super fillings" and the power of the Holy Spirit.

The message long past due is JOHN'S message of preparation. The most important message of this day (as before Jesus' first advent), is John's message, PRE-PARE and make your paths straight. The message of this hour is John's message. It is the mesage that will get people ready for a big event. It is a warning message; it is the last message, and the vital message of the hour. John's message has to do with Jesus and His Kingdom. If God's people will heed this message it will kill the old carnal nature, and put man in his proper place in respect to spiritual things. John's message has to do with the perfecting of God's people, it is the refining message. It is the message that deals WITH THE PLAIN SIMPLE WAY OF LIVING, SIMPLE DRESS AND ATTIRE; A PLAIN SIMPLE MENU with PLENTY OF FAST-INGS TO ALWAYS KEEP THE APPETITES WHOLLY YIELDED TO GOD.

The truth concerning fasting was very prominently taught by John the Baptist. He did not care whether the people liked it or not. John hewed to the line. He beat out the flesh and stamped upon it. He was making his appearance to God and not to man. Jesus Christ said that "He was the greatest man born of woman," because he fasted often and kept the flesh down. That is why it cost him his life. The message of John was to God's people, a message of fasting and prayer. The message of fasting and prayer is likewise the final message to God's saints to wake up and make their final preparation for His coming again. (See Joel, first and second chapters).

The answer to JOHN'S DISCIPLES was, "When the bridegroom shall be taken away from them, then shall they FAST." Matt. 9:15. This should settle permanently any doubt concerning when we should fast or whether or not we should wait until God lays a fasting burden upon us. JESUS has already settled the question. "THEN shall they fast." Did the BRIDEGROOM leave us? If He did, then we are to fast. There should be no further argument

about it. Many Scriptures show us that it is more important to fast now than at any other time, lest we be
asleep and "that day come upon us unawares". Luke 21:
34. Matt. 24:38.

Jesus also told His followers something else that
should take place after He went away. "It is expedient
for you that I go away: for if I go not away, the Com-
forter will not come unto you; but if I depart, I will send
him unto you." John 16:7. Yes, the Bridegroom left so
that the Spirit of truth could come if His disciples and
followers would prepare to receive Him. Again just before
He ascended He told them: "Ye shall receive power, after
that the Holy Ghost is come upon you." Acts 1:8. Jesus
again emphasizes the importance of the Holy Spirit when
He "Commanded them that they should not depart from
Jerusalem, but wait for the promise of the Father, which,
saith he, ye have heard of me." Acts 1:4.

It is very evident that the one-hundred-twenty who
tarried in the upper room also remembered something else
that the Bridegroom told them they would do when He
would be taken away, and this something was that they
would FAST. Their hearts being grieved and saddened at
the loss of the Bridegroom, of course they would obey HIM.
This is very likely what they were doing when they were
"Continuing with one accord in prayer and supplication."
Consequently they received the super-dynamic FILLING
of the Holy Ghost and Fire that literally shook the whole
city and country and affected the whole world.

Why do we not fulfil all of the requirements of Jesus
Christ nowadays? "If a man love me, he will keep my
words: and my Father will love him, and we will come
unto him, and make our abode with him." John 14:23.

I am not trying to leave the impression that it is
necessary to fast in order to receive the Baptism of the
Holy Spirit. However, the divine manifestation in the
upper room appears to have been far greater than in the
many tarrying meetings nowadays where people also receive the Baptism of the Holy Spirit but not in quite the
same super atomic manner.

I have seen many a Christian pray and tarry for the
Holy Spirit for many months and not receive Him. They
did not seem to be putting their all into it. Finally they
became more in earnest and started a fast with their

prayers, and soon they received the blessed Spirit.

This was the experience of the author. Many times for over two years the Holy Spirit was sought without results. I was frequently discouraged and it seemed it was of no use. In desperation I began seeking God more earnestly, however, until nothing mattered but God. Yes, I finally wanted the Holy Spirit more than I wanted to eat. Many meals were omitted, and for days I was lost in God in prayer and fasting. After only about eight days of this, the Lord gloriously filled me with His Holy Spirit.

This same method is also applicable to the receiving of your HEALING or the answer to any prayer you may be praying.

The women were also in the upper room instead of at home cooking meals. "They continued in one accord in prayer and supplication." In "continuing" in this one accord, it is doubtful if they had time to run around buying up groceries, or going back and forth, carrying on all the other details connected with the cooking and preparing of meals, as well as the washing and cleaning up after eating.

Most Bible teachers will agrere with me that the believers prayed and fasted while tarrying in the upper room.

PRAYERS ANSWERED THROUGH FASTING IN CANADA

Dear Brother Hall:

I always believed in fasting and prayer but didn't know how to fast ten days or longer until I got to studying the Bible along with your writings.

After fasting over ten days, I received much spiritual help and I had more understanding of the Bible that I ever had, as well as prayers answered.

Please send some literature to Pastor ....

Sincerely yours,

E. H.

St. John

N. B. Canada

Chapter III

THE REFINING FIRE OF PERFECTION

DOWN WITH THE FLESH

Galatians 5:13-25: "For, brethren, ye have been called unto liberty; only USE NOT LIBERTY FOR AN OCCASION TO THE FLESH, . . . Walk in the Spirit, and ye shall not fulfill the lust of the flesh. FOR THE FLESH LUSTETH AGAINST THE SPIRIT, and the SPIRIT AGAINST the FLESH: and these are contrary the one to the other: so that ye cannot do the things that ye would.

"Now the works of the flesh are manifest, which are these;

Adultery	**Fornication**
Uncleanness	**Lasciviousness**
Idolatry	**Witchcraft**
Hatred	**Variance**
Emulations	**Wrath**
Strife	**Seditions**
Heresies	**Envyings**
Murders	**Drunkenness**
Revellings	**and such like:**

of the which I tell you before, as I have also told you in time past, that they which do such things shall not inherit the kingdom of God.

"But the FRUIT of the Spirit is love, joy, peace, long-suffering, gentleness, goodness, faith, meekness, temperance: against such there is no law. And they that are Christ's have CRUCIFIED THE FLESH with the affections and lusts."

Gal. 6:8: "For he that soweth to his FLESH SHALL OF THE FLESH REAP CORRUPTION; but he that soweth to the Spirit shall of the Spirit reap LIFE EVERLASTING."

The above listed "works of the flesh" are also men-

tioned in duplication in Colossians 3:5. Paul calls it "the
course of this world" in Ephesians 2:2. These are also "the
LUSTS OF OUR FLESH", "THE DESIRES OF THE
FLESH" Eph. 2:3. It would be more easily understood
if we just called the "LUSTS" and "DESIRES OF THE
FLESH" abnormal or over-developed appetites. I have
made a careful study of the APPETITES and I have found
that man has only four major NATURAL APPETITES.
They are HUNGER, SEX, THE COVETOUS APPE-
TITE GREED and the SPIRITUAL. These appetites are
normal and natural when the SPIRITUAL APPETITE
is predominant, and is developed by spiritual things as
the WORDS OF GOD and by PRAYER AND FAST-
INGS. When our spiritual appetite is neglected it becomes
dwarfed into insignificance, and the other three appetites
grow abnormally out of all proportion. These three natural
appetites that are always giving us trouble in the flesh,
and which will help to make up the "old man" that wars
against the spirit, and makes the soul the battleground,
are always breaking faith unexpectedly somewhere. The
appetites, and sense faculties, which are centered in the
appetites, help to make up the old man and carnality.
This is why we should always be prayed up and FAST
OFTEN to keep them in subjection, and by proper eating
they can stay "MORTIFIED".

Each of these works of the flesh is traceable directly
to one or more of our appetites. In fact, each can be seg-
regated so it will fall into one of the three groups.

It has been established by both medical science and
spiritually minded persons that the HUNGER APPE-
TITE, as well as being the most powerful of the three
appetites, also holds the key to the temperance or intemperance of the other two carnal appetites of SEX and
GREED. Perhaps I have expressed it stronger than they
do by stating the HUNGER APPETITE FEEDS the
other two.

There are many kinds of hunger. If one can abolish
the food HUNGER, he can become empty enough to permit his spiritual appetite to crave, thirst, and hunger to a
much greater degree after the things of God. He may have
a greater hunger to see souls born into the kingdom. If
he does not have the Holy Spirit and begins seeking for

Him, he will find that hunger satisfied in the filling or re-filling of the Spirit. He may hunger to see God's power manifested in healings and miracles. If the candidate becomes burdened for the same, he will see them come to pass through fasting. He could bear a financial burden for God's work, or many other deep hunger burdens. Maybe it will be only one, and it could be many.

"Blessed are they which do hunger and thirst after righteousness; FOR THEY SHALL BE FILLED." Matt. 5:6.

Generally speaking, when I mention hunger in this volume, I refer to "FOOD HUNGER." The real hunger that is present in this appetite gives a zest for food to nourish one's body. However this hunger appetite may be divided into three phases.

(1). TRUE HUNGER.

This hunger usually leaves, in fasting, by the fourth day. True, real hunger returns in a complete fast in from 21 to 40 days or longer.

(2).HABIT HUNGER.

When a whistle blows, or when a certain time arrives, a person eats. A certain habit in eating is acquired, whether the individual has a real appetite for the food he eats or not, therefore the eating habit is formed. Habit hunger shows up frequently in fasting, especially during the first part of the fast. It may be present off and on throughout the entire fast. It usually appears around meal time but could appear at any time. It usually can be abolished by keeping the mind on the Lord, and it could be difficult to dismiss from one's mind.

(3). THE HUNGER OF THE OTHER APPETITES.

Because of the fact that the appetites of carnality are not under stimulation from the use of food (and they are fed or derive their power from food), they in turn cause the individual to feel laxed and undone, thereby reminding the faster that food is necessary to have that good feeling of worldly satisfaction and enjoyment he desires. This hunger is present through-

out the fast, though to a lesser degree after about
two weeks. Many times these different hungers are
confused with one another.

After several weeks of the fast, and the proper breaking in to eating, which is very important in order not to
overstimulate the natural appetites, our spiritual appetite
or nature is so highly developed by the FASTING
PRAYER one finds it easier to keep "UNDER MY
BODY." It has been brought "INTO SUBJECTION."
See I Cor. 9:25-27. The proper "MASTERY . . . IN ALL
THINGS" can be held as long as the KEY to it all, which
is proper eating and deep consecration to Jesus Christ, is
maintained. Too often, however, we mingle with the crowd
or have some tempting dinner engagements, and we yield to
the hunger temptation and our appetite, before we are
aware, becomes abnormal. Another fast, or strict abstemious living will then be necessary to bring us back to the
straight and narrow way so Jesus Christ can be greatly
glorified.

THE GREAT WARFARE

The Bible tells from beginning to end of the GREAT
WARFARE BETWEEN THE FLESH AND THE
SPIRIT, a fight between the APPETITES of man and
his SPIRITUAL PROGRESS, a battle between good and
evil, between the natural and the spiritual, between the
earthly and the heavenly, between the lower forces and
the higher, between the corruptible and the incorruptible,
between intemperance and temperance, between filthiness
and cleanness, between haughtiness and humility, between
the proud and the meek, between selfishness and selfless-
ness, between carnality and the supernatural, and between
the OLD MAN AND THE NEW MAN. All of the evils
may be traced to the FLESH.

The FLESH gets in the way, perhaps more than any
other obstacle, in the prevention of God's dealing with
mankind in the manner in which He would be pleased.
The old flesh, by hindering our faith, prevents our secur-
ing the answers to our prayers. Our healing, and many
other beautiful experiences we should have had from the
throne of God long ago are painfully denied to us because
the OLD MAN OF FLESH has never been sufficiently

subdued for God, Who is always willing, to give us "the desire of our heart."

The Word of God is full of accounts of the weaknesses and failures of the flesh which have prevented many victories from getting through to His people.

Paul continually emphasized the value of keeping the flesh under subjugation. He beat down his own flesh, he hammered at it constantly, and kept it subdued by "FASTINGS OFTEN" II Cor. 11:27. It was very important to Paul that he should "KEEP UNDER MY BODY, and bring it into subjugation: lest that by any means, when I have preached to others, I myself should be a castaway." 1 Cor. 9:27. Paul is talking definitely about proper eating and living. This is the best way to keep the appetite lusts under control. So important is abstemious living for God's people that Paul tells about a special reward to be given to those who live thus. "EVERY MAN THAT STRIVETH FOR THE MASTERY IS TEMPERATE IN ALL THINGS. Many practice temperance to obtain a corruptible crown; but WE AN INCORRUPTIBLE. I THEREFORE SO RUN, NOT AS UNCERTAINLY; SO FIGHT I, NOT AS ONE THAT BEATETH THE AIR; BUT I KEEP MY BODY UNDER. (FLESH UNDER CONTROL)" 1 Cor. 9:25-27.

THE FIVE CROWNS

Paul well knew the value of keeping the appetite "UNDER" control so this great reward of the "INCORRUPTIBLE CROWN" could be attained. Too many people are running this part of their race with uncertainty. They say, "What difference does it make whether I FAST TEN DAYS OR NOT, or what difference does it make what I eat, when I eat, how often I eat or how much I eat—I will do as I please about eating, ask God's blessing on it, and let it go at that." So they do as they choose and satisfy completely their appetites. But the Word of God is sure, and the rewards and judgments certainly will come to pass regardless of those who let their lusts run wide open, whether it pertains to food or other appetites of the flesh.

Paul emphasizes the fact he was not just beating the air, not knowing what he was doing, but he was "STRIV-

ING," he was laboring with difficulty, to run that he might have this special reward. Indeed it is with labor that anyone must strive to live right, and eat properly, as well as fast and pray that he may keep this old fleshly body "UNDER."

This very precious reward will be given only to those who keep the flesh "MORTIFIED." See Col. 3:5. Mortification means abstinence, and this is most effective by fasting, at least occassionally, and eating right, so the food babies will get the upper hand. (See chart elsewhere on this subject.)

There will be a special crowning day when the rewards will be given to all of God's saints who will keep the "BODY UNDER" subjugation. This *incorruptible crown* is one of the five special crowns that will be given to those who "RUN THAT WE MAY OBTAIN" (our good works). This presentation will take place on the crowning day at the JUDGMENT SEAT OF CHRIST when final judgment is passed upon the saints for the works done in the body after Christ has been accepted as Saviour. (1 Cor. 3:13-15.) I mention them so as to bring to our attention the fact that we should strive more earnestly to receive them. Fasting and prayer, as well as temperate living, will also enable us more easily to receive these other glorious CROWNS. The five CROWNS are:

1. The crown of RIGHTEOUSNESS FOR THOSE THAT LOVE HIS APPEARING. 11 Tim. 4:8.

2. The crown of REJOICING, a SOUL WINNER'S CROWN. 1 Thes. 2:19.

3. The crown of GLORY, the pastor, worker, or shepherd's CROWN. 1 Pet. 5:4.

4. The MARTYR'S CROWN for those FAITHFUL UNTO DEATH. Rev. 2:10.

5. AN INCORRUPTIBLE CROWN. 1 Cor. 9:25-27. (The CROWN under consideration.)

"Now they do it to obtain a corruptible crown; but we an INCORRUPTIBLE. I therefore so run, not as uncertainly; so fight I, not as one that beateth the air: But

I keep under my body, AND BRING IT INTO SUBJEC-
TION: LEST THAT BY ANY MEANS, WHEN I HAVE
PREACHED TO OTHERS, I MYSELF SHOULD BE
A CASTAWAY." Even Paul realized that he would not
obtain this great reward if he did not go after it with his
whole heart. He realized he might be a "castaway," or
lose this great reward. This would not mean, however,
that he would fail of salvation if he did not receive the
reward. I am sure we would like to strive more earnestly
to secure everything it is possible to obtain, and to glorify
our blessed Redeemer who gave His all, and shed His blood
for us so we might have eternal life. This fact should
inspire us to work with all our might, and to be the best
that we can for our Lord. "Present your BODIES a
LIVING SACRIFICE, holy, acceptable unto God, which
is your reasonable service. And be not conformed to this
world: but be ye transformed by the renewing of your
mind, that ye may prove what is good, and acceptable,
and perfect, will of God." Rom. 12:1, 2. The presentation
of the body as a living sacrifice for the praise and honor of
Jesus Christ can best be accomplished through FASTING
AND PRAYER. One way in which this LIVING SACRI-
FICE can be offered is through the giving up of food for
a time and living the fasted life. Although there are
other ways of making our bodies a living sacrifice, I would
be happy to know which of them could be more effective
than to go into a FASTING PRAYER once in a while for
the glory of God. Whatever the method employed to
present our bodies a living sacrifice, the Scripture further
states it is a "REASONABLE SERVICE." Whatever the
sacrifice, and whatever the cost may be, even if it is FAST-
ING, it will be a low price to pay to be fully "ACCEP-
TABLE UNTO GOD." Fasting is a method of "RENEW-
ING THE MIND." I have personally seen it work like
magic. I have seen talkative individuals who had difficulty
in bridling their tongues, go on a fast and have their minds
so renewed that they acquired control of the unruly member. Some hot heads who were afflicted with fiery tempers
have come out from fasts with their minds fully "renewed."
Fasting helps to remove jealousies, evil thoughts, hatred,
malice, pride, and many other things which come from
the mind which needs "renewing" through FASTING AND

PRAYER. This acts as a refining fire. It gets rid of dross.

1 Cor. 10:31: "Whether therefore ye eat, or drink, or whatsoever ye do, DO ALL TO THE GLORY OF GOD." If as shown by medical statistics, the great majority of sicknesses are caused by wrong eating and overeating, how can we GLORIFY GOD when we eat food our bodies do not need? If our bodies do not require the full amount of food we eat, we will be stimulating the carnal appetites, and this will be one cause for failure to GLORIFY GOD THE WAY WE SHOULD. In other words, overeating feeds the fleshy lusts and causes imperfections.

KING OVER THE FLESH

If we do not master the flesh, the flesh will master us. FASTING is a "BLITZKRIEG" set up for the subjugation of the flesh. There is no more rapid, efficient, or effective way to carry on warfare against the flesh than through the FASTING PRAYER. This will bring perfection, which in turn will enable us to receive spiritual gifts.

FASTING will greatly aid in the "CRUCIFYING OF THE FLESH." Rom. 6:6. "Our old man is CRUCIFIED with Him, that the body of sin might be destroyed, that henceforth we should not serve sin." In the NEW BIRTH the believer has already been reckoned with, and he is here exhorted to make good this new experience. Gal. 5:24: "They that are Christ's have crucified the flesh with the affections and lusts." Fasting will aid in keeping the old man crucified, so our CONSECRATION will be fully complete before the Lord. The flesh is deceitful, and at times we do not know we are actually slipping in our experience with God. Many Christians who were once on fire for God have grown cold, and the strange thing about it is they do not realize it. Paul warns of this when he gives the exhortation to "Be renewed in the spirit of your mind." Eph. 4:23. WHY? Because, "Ye put off concerning the former conversation the old man, which is corrupt according to THE DECEITFUL LUSTS." Plan to have regular periods of the FASTING PRAYER in your life, and you will have a Christian experience that will dominate the flesh, and a reign of spiritual power in your life. Then your life will be a "living sacrifice" to THE GLORY OF GOD.

Here is a testimony of a precious brother who did

whip the flesh into line, not by just a few days of fasting, but he fasted forty days and his spirit was KING over the flesh so that God mightily used him (see his book for more details):

> "I have fasted many times in my life and have taken some big fasts. I have had many revelations and visions as a result of these fasts. Some of these visions concerned the 'resurrection,' others pertained to the 'end of the world,' and many concerned 'prophecy.' I have always received something very valuable from every protracted fast that I have ever been in. VICTORY HAS ALWAYS COME.
>
> "As I have related in my life story, not so many years ago, and with only about seventy-five dollars to my name, the Lord called me to go to a certain city in the southeastern part of the United States and *FAST for forty days.* Immediately following that fast, A REVIVAL BROKE OUT THERE IN WHICH OVER SEVEN THOUSAND WENT TO AN OLD-FASHIONED ALTAR AND CONFESSED JESUS CHRIST AS THEIR LORD AND SAVIOR, and over two thousand were healed of all manner of diseases and infirmities through the gift of healing."
>
> R. M. Smith
> Box 729
> Pasadena, Calif.

The greatest enemy of the Christian is the flesh. "HAVE NO CONFIDENCE IN THE FLESH." Phil. 3:3. The flesh prevents more of God's children from having what He wills for them, than anything else. It is leaned upon far more than anyone can imagine or think possible; deadens faith, and prevents one from believing the promises and getting answers from God. Jesus plainly shows us UNBELIEF is a work of the flesh, otherwise why would he tell us that faith as a grain of mustard seed would remove mountains, and cometh only "By PRAYER AND FASTING," as recorded in Matthew, chapter 17? The reason for this is plainly evident. The flesh must be whipped into line before we can have the mountain-removing FAITH, and this is a product of FASTING, which will subdue the flesh more efficiently than anything else. If not, why did Jesus give us this process?

The flesh and the Spirit of God are as far apart in their relationship to each other as East is from West. They do not get along, and they never will. Let us see the flesh defeated more often through the FASTING PRAYER.

"The FLESH LUSTETH *AGAINST* THE SPIRIT, and the SPIRIT *AGAINST* THE FLESH." As soon as we become converted a major BATTLE begins. This is a WARFARE against the FLESH and "NOT AFTER THE FLESH:" (11 Cor. 10:3--5). "For though we walk in the FLESH, we do not WAR AFTER THE FLESH." "The weapons of our warfare are not carnal, but MIGHTY THROUGH GOD to the pulling down of strong-holds." Thank God for our SPIRITUAL WEAPONS TO AID US IN THE FIGHT. At times the fight is terrific, but these spiritual weapons are available to us in whatever manner we need them, and they come as powerful as is necessary to defeat the enemy. A large quantity of this spiritual equipment will be at our command through fasting and prayer. With God on our side there is nothing to fear.

While this great warfare goes on, there is great turmoil within the soul because the soul is the BATTLE-GROUND between the FLESH AND THE SPIRIT. When the Spirit comes out VICTOR there is not only a "HOLDING FAITH WITH A GOOD CONSCIENCE," but there is new faith gained in the battle. 1 Tim. 1:18,19: "That thou mightest WAR a good WARFARE; HOLD-ING FAITH, and a good conscience; which some having put away concerning faith have made shipwreck:" We do not stand still in our Christian experience but we are progressive. "We run."

If the flesh should be victorious in this spiritual conflict, the soul will still be the battleground, but one's FAITH will have been "shipwrecked."

The mastery of the flesh is a continous FIGHT. At times it may be a hotter fight than at other times, but it will always be a fight as long as the body is the temple and abiding place of the precious Holy Spirit.

1 Cor. 6:19,20: "Know ye not that your body is the temple of the Holy Ghost which is in you, which ye have of God, and ye are NOT YOUR OWN? FOR YE ARE BOUGHT WITH A PRICE: THEREFORE GLORIFY GOD IN YOUR *BODY*, AND IN YOUR SPIRIT, WHICH ARE GOD'S."

Prayer and deep consecration will GLORIFY GOD, but at times we should go further. THE MOST EFFECTIVE WAY TO DO THIS IS THROUGH THE FASTING PRAYER. This will keep down the flesh, and both spirit and body can be a sweet aroma for the glory of God.

Following the above Scripture, and in the same letter to the Corinthian church, Paul gave some further instruction concerning the FASTING PRAYER. In the sixth and seventh chapters of Paul's first letter to the Corinthians, he gave certain teachings concerning the SANCTITY OF THE BODY AND MARRIAGE. This concerned the members of the body which are, after all, the members of Christ. This was in relationship to the control of the flesh and the proper subjugation of the appetites.

To the married couple, Paul said, "Defraud ye not one the other, except it be with consent for a TIME, that ye may give yourselves to FASTING AND PRAYER; and come together again, that Satan tempt you not for your INCONTINENCE." 1 Cor. 7:5.

If one partner wanted to go into a protracted fast long enough to inconvenience the other partner through denial of the marriage relationship, consent of the opposite partner should be obtained. When a partner goes into this protracted season of prayer and fasting, as has previously been pointed out, there will not be the desire of the natural appetites after a few days; they will have been surrendered through food abstention, so the SPIRITUAL APPETITE WILL BE ENLARGED TO SUPER CAPACITY FOR THE GREAT THINGS DESIRED FROM GOD. Any effort to satisfy any one of the carnal appetites at this time, while in the FASTING PRAYER, whether it is through the appetite of hunger, sex, or that of covetousness, will mitigate and retard the fasting candidate's efforts to break through to the desired success in the VICTORIOUS "FAST THROUGH" EXPERIENCE.

I do not believe Paul meant that it would be sinful for a couple to indulge their appetites while one or the other was in a fast, but I feel the spiritual results that might be obtained, will have been retarded, therefore one should secure permission beforehand for the "TIME" of "FASTING AND PRAYER" so there may be no interruption in the days or weeks of fasting, before God which belongs to Him. (Paul speaks this by permission). In this Scripture it may be observed the "TIME" of fasting referred to did not mean a short fast of several meals, but referred to a protracted fast of a number of days. It probably referred to an important fast perhaps a major fast of ten days or longer. If it referred only to a short fast, there would be no need to obtain special permission of each other for complete abstinence. At that time some of the couples had friction and trouble with one another. To avoid having controversy, obtain permission from each other. (Please study Joel 2:15, 16, along this line.)

After the great victory of prayer and fasting, "come together again." The physical and spiritual purification that goes on, through the fast, and through the subjugation of the appetites for "TIME," so cleanse and purify the creative forces that this time is a most auspicious season to attract a soul which would be born nine months later under ideal SPIRITUAL conditions. This deep consecration to God would insure the parent of such a lofty spiritual environment in which to bring forth children that God would bless his offspring in an unusual manner. Experiences along this line have proved this to be true.

Samuel was a product of a consecrated fast by his mother Hannah. (1 Samuel Chapter I.)

Reverend Jack Walker tells of a FASTING experience along this line:

> "Twelve years ago I was having a great spiritual battle. I set my face to FASTING AND PRAYER in sackcloth and ashes, like Daniel. I was severely criticized, scorned, made fun of, and they even 'shaked their heads' at me like they did at David. Sad to say, some religious leaders even belittled my efforts in my humble manner of seeking God.

"I sought God very earnestly in fasting for FOURTEEN days. At the conclusion of this fast the soul of LITTLE DAVID was attracted and given to my wife and me. Nine months later he was born. He began to be used mightily of God, under the anointing of the Spirit, at the age of only nine. He is twelve now, and God has given him thousands of souls, and he has spoken from coast to coast in the largest city auditoriums available. Thousands of people have been prayed for and healed, thank God.

"At the age of nine, Little David's spirit left his body while fasting five days. He says, 'I spent five hours in Heaven. Jesus sent me to preach.'

"Many other things happened in answer to prayer at the conclusion of this fast. I prayed for an epileptic person, and the demons were immediately cast out and the man was made whole. Other major healings took place in answer to prayer and as a result of this fast.

"In St. Louis, Missouri, I had one of the largest meetings of my life. Many souls were saved and large crowds were moved by the power of the Spirit. Praise the Lord for ever.

"Fasting is continually practiced in our meetings, and God always hears and answers prayers by giving us many souls and by healing the sick. Fasting is seriously needed in the Church of Jesus Christ today so that miracles and the gifts can be restored to make the BRIDE of Christ all she ought to be."

Jack Walker.

SIX FAST TWENTY-ONE DAYS AND 600 CONVERTED

Four members of our evangelistic party went to Indianapolis while fasting twenty-one days without any food. They gave talks on fasting to the church people in behalf of a revival. The Christians were so amazed to see people on a fast from fourteen to twenty days, (the length of time on the twenty-one day fast) they were also provoked

to start fasting. Brother Raymond Hoekstra's church secured four hundred revival books, "Atomic Power With
God Through Fasting and Prayer," and fifty folk were
left fasting for a revival.

Thirty days later, July 20, 1947, the greatest revival
that ever came to Indianapolis was in progress in Cadle
Tabernacle which seats 10,000. It was packed with 11,000
people, and one thousand turned away.

In one service alone, two hundred-fifty sinners came
forward weeping their way to Jesus. At least six hundred
came to an old fashion altar in this great FASTING
PRAYER campaign. Many testified to being healed instantly.

Two other members of our party, including myself,
fasted twenty-one days, three fasted ten days and one
twelve days. Little David (12 year old boy preacher)
fasted five days. This was our first meeting after the fast.

The FASTING PRAYER, which is the consecration
fast to the Christian, will surrender, put the flesh under
subjection and empty out all of the fleshly carnal nature
of the old man so the NEW MAN can operate to the
fullest extent in the manner the Holy Spirit wishes. This
is, of course, to EXALT JESUS CHRIST and let HIM
reign supreme in our lives so new praises of joy, thanksgiving, and deep spiritual consecration can rush forth as
fountains of water from within our souls. While in this
different kind of prayer which is so successful in praising
and honoring HIM whom our soul loveth, we at times
are lost in a new realm of spiritual environment that
overshadows anything we have heretofore experienced.
After victory we feel so light we would like to leave this
old world and at times feel as though we could be translated at any moment. After a complete "fast through"
experience in the fasting prayer, and if the individual
has the Holy Spirit, there is no greater joy or satisfaction
to be reached in human experience than that which is
obtainable while in this body on a major fast. It is the
"de-luxe" of spiritual experiences sublime.

THE HUMAN STORAGE BATTERY

The average physical body contains two million live
cells. These two million cells when functioning normally
are magnetic and electric in their relationship to each

other, and to the various functional organs of the body. They radiate life, and act just as one great storage battery to make health and physical life complete. The food one eats keeps these wonderful cells fully charged up and ready for activity. Very often they become "overcharged." When overcharged they become choked up and inefficient. The magnetism is lost, and if this choked up condition is continued through more food indulgences and "OVERCHARGING," a food bulge is the result. This food bulge shows up in the body in a manner similar to the way an inner tube appears when too much air is pumped into it and it forms a bulge on one side. Sometimes a FOOD BULGE assumes a shape similar to the shape and appearance of the air bulge seen in an over-inflated inner tube or old tire. The over-inflated stomach or the "overcharged" stomach, as Jesus Christ calls it in Luke 21:34, forms a food bulge somewhere in the body and maybe it is called a TUMOR. A food bulge is also called a cyst, an obnoxious growth, a goitre, or some other affliction that may be nothing more than an OVERCHARGED condition of some of these two million cells.

Because we are leaving the Piscian age, and are entering the Aquarian age, which is the machine age of speed, and which brings a host of evil influences along with it, we may now look for greater expressions of the lower passions, such as alamentiveness or over-eating and drinking, and its natural correlary amativeness. Other expressions of the lower passions as combativeness, destruction, and lack of natural affection will be the order of the day.

Jesus warns of this condition, and wherever the laws of God are disobeyed, man is certain to reap the consequences, whether or not it be from the sin of over-eating or some other sin which may seem worse, but in reality is not.

Luke 21:34: "Take heed (this means WARNING) to yourselves, lest at any time your hearts be *OVERCHARGED with surfeiting,* and drunkenness, and cares of this life, and so THAT DAY COME UPON YOU UNAWARES. For as a snare shall it come on all them that dwell on the face of the whole earth. WATCH ye therefore, AND PRAY *ALWAYS,* that ye may be accounted worthy to escape all these things that shall come to pass,

and to stand before the Son of man." SURFEITING:
(definition) AN OVERLOADING OF THE STOMACH
BY EXCESS IN EATING; A GLUTTONOUS MEAL.
When the stomach becomes overloaded, the cells become
polluted and the food bulge, or some other malady that
may be either milder or more severe, is the result. The
two million cells no more vibrate with health magnetism,
but a serious condition is the result which affects our spiritual welfare. This is nothing more than the lusts of the
flesh being abnormally indulged through the three or
even four MEAL A DAY STUFFING HABIT.   The
little faith we might have had becomes stifled, and the
flesh is on the loose, with carnality seeking some form
of outlet. If prayer, or prayer and fasting is not entered
upon the person may be on the verge of slipping away
from the "FAITH THAT HE ONCE HAD."

Unconsciously, too many folk almost get to worshiping
food and don't realize it. An over-emphasis is placed on
its value and it ranks ahead of everything else. Jesus
makes it clear what He thinks of the condition that will
prevail everywhere in the last days! Paul shows how little
food matters to him when he says, "Meats for the BELLY,
AND the BELLY FOR MEATS: but God shall DES-
TROY BOTH IT AND THEM." 1 Cor. 6:13.

These two million cells are as definitely charged with
nourishment as the cells of a battery are kept charged by
a generator. These cellular tissues can be "OVERCHARG-
ED with SURFEITING," as JESUS CALLS IT, just as
easily as a storage battery can become overcharged on
the car you drive when it does not have a voltage control regulator between the generator and the battery. A
number of years ago automobiles did not have a storage
battery regulator to cut off automatically the excess
current and prevent overcharging of the battery. Consequently, many a battery was ruined prematurely. Today most cars have an automatic regulator which prevents
damage to the battery through the generation of too much
electricity from the generator into its CELLS. Too much
charging depletes the cells, breaks them down prematurely,
overheats them or causes them to deteriorate in a short
time. The cells which make up the storage battery can
no longer accept the charge of electricity. Sometimes, if

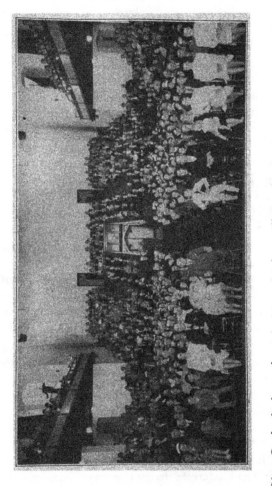

The Scottish-Rite Cathedral at the tri-cities, Moline, Ill. A fasting-prayer revival. Afternoon services were held in the Presbyterian Church. The Methodist, Baptist, Christians, United Brethern, Nazarine, Lutheran and many churches cooperated with us in a city wide campaign. Our entire party occupies the entire front row.

it has not been overcharged too much, and ruined completely, the battery will hold a partial charge, but even
then it will last for only a very short time.

Many an individual who bears the name of Christ
has his own two million cells so overcharged with SUR-
FEITING that he is suffering with some affliction that
is due to nothing more than his intemperate eating. This
causes a pollution of the blood stream and the cellular
tissues through the introduction, development and accumulation of toxins fermentation, debris, putrefaction,
or other waste matter within the physical system, to such
an extent that the ordinary physiological processes of
elimination can no longer handle it in the normal and
regular way of EXCRETION. In addition to the sicknesses
or afflictions that come about through these fleshly sins
of surfeiting, frequently, the other appetites turn into
some form of fleshly lust, and much difficulty (sometimes
unconsciously acquired) is experienced in the spiritual
life. The consecration is weakened and one does not have
a LIVING VICTORIOUS EXPERIENCE OF FAITH
BEFORE GOD. Often these SURFEITERS wonder why
they are not getting anywhere with God. The reason is
very evident. Just as soon as there is an abstention from
eating, these two million cells prove themselves just as
inherently capable of sustaining the life (without more
food) as the battery is able to continue giving forth
electricity for service without the generator continuing with
its charge. The food acts as a generator to the human body.
These cells can go on without food for not only days but
weeks, and in this process there is a cessation not only
of self-pollution and self-poisoning but an opportunity for
the overtaxed eliminative processes to begin HOUSE-
CLEANING. THE STOMACH HAS A HOLIDAY.
THESE TWO MILLION CELLS ARE AT LAST GIVEN
A VACATION. The system has been so overloaded by
SURFEITING and the accumulation of material that
the vital energies cannot always keep up the laborious
task of digesting, converting, and pushing food material
through the THIRTY FEET of tubing efficiently as they
should. The OVERCHARGED CELLS block the circulation of blood, and become so choked up that these cells
which should function and perform for the glory of God,
are no longer radiating with vibrating magnetism to aid

in keeping the FLESHLY LUSTS UNDER SUBJEC-
TION, but become perverted, and God has to turn his
back upon the individual for the time being.

What is the answer? A FASTING PRAYER is the
quickest way to solve the problem. It will not only reno-
vate these many cells by restoring them to new invigorat-
ing particles of life, but the whole fleshly nature, including
all of the natural appetites, will have had such a reno-
vating and clearing away of the filthy flesh of the "OLD
MAN" it will be like a rug just returned from the cleaners.
The rug was old looking, dirty, spotted and wrinkled. It
was taken, and shaken, and rolled around and around;
it was beaten, stirred up, shampooed with cleaning materials, and pressed. When the rug was returned it was clean
and beautiful, and the old colors were restored in the
process. When a person goes into a protracted season of
prayer and fasting, it sometimes seems like we are about
to die, and the old flesh really takes a beating, a pounding,
and a cleaning. At times we seems to be going down into
despair and feel God has forgotten us. This is nothing more
that a complete renovation and house cleaning of the OLD
MAN and it will work out ultimately for the great and
grand GLORY of our SAVIOUR JESUS CHRIST.
AMEN! Why should we not be happy to go through a few
trials and tribulations if you want to call FASTING that?
The results are worth while and much to be desired.
Think of it, the eradication of the very things the OLD
MAN doesn't want eradicated is not only the best thing for
us spiritually but it is also gloriously beneficial for us
physically. It not only will make us live longer, but will
enable us to live the more ABUNDANT LIFE for the
praise and glory of JESUS.

The voltage regulator for the storage battery automatically prevents the "OVERSTUFFING" by electricity
of the cells that make up the battery. The life of the battery is more than doubled by this safety measure.
Human beings have no automatic regulator control to
prevent "OVERSTUFFING" and "OVERCHARGING"
of the cellular tissues. When a sinner becomes converted,
he "WALKS NOT AFTER THE FLESH, BUT AFTER
THE SPIRIT. For they that are after the flesh do mind
the things of the flesh: but they that are after the Spirit
the things of the Spirit. For to be CARNALLY minded

is death; but to be spiritually minded is life and peace. Because the *CARNAL mind is enmity against God*: for it is not subject to the law of God, neither indeed can be. They that are in THE FLESH CANNOT PLEASE GOD. BUT YE ARE NOT IN THE FLESH, but in the SPIRIT, if so be that the Spirit of God dwell in you." Romans 8:4-9. As children of God we do have the Holy Spirit to lead us, but too often we do not stay close enough to God in FASTING AND PRAYER to be able to hear the gentle voice of the Spirit, and He is GRIEVED away so far that we go on in *OUR OWN will* rather than in the directive will of the Spirit. We would rather please ourselves, which is nothing more than gratification of the desires of the FLESH, than to wait on the Spirit. Even though we may not stay close enough always to hear the Spirit speak to us, or to know He is grieved with our intemperance and "OVERCHARGING," we do have the PLAIN SIMPLE TEACHINGS OF JESUS IN THE WORD OF GOD TO GUIDE US IN THIS REGARD. THERE CAN BE NO EXCUSE FOR FAILING TO EAT RIGHT AND LIVE THE SIMPLE LIFE AS WELL AS FAST AND FAST OFTEN. The above Scripture in Romans has enough truth-revealing factors in it alone to induce one to follow the SPIRIT *and not to be* "DEBTORS TO THE FLESH, to LIVE AFTER THE FLESH." Please take heed, and study the seventh and eighth chapters of Romans. Both the Word of God and the precious HOLY SPIRIT can EFFECTIVELY REGULATE THE WAY WE LIVE IF WE LET OUR FLESHLY WILL BE CONQUERED BY SAYING YES TO GOD AND NO TO OUR DESIRES. The Holy Spirit then becomes our regulator.

FASTING PREVENTS DIVISIONS

> "*Mark* them which cause divisions and offences contrary to the doctrine which ye have learned; and *avoid* them. For they that are such serve not our Lord Jesus Christ, BUT THEIR OWN BELLY; and by good words and fair speeches deceive the hearts of the simple." Rom. 16:17, 18.

A person cannot have a twisted inharmonious under-

standing of the Word of God when taking regular protracted seasons of fastings. Fasting gives one the correct
interpretation of the scriptures. It will remove by revelation any lopsided petty issue that may have been
incorrectly interpreted previous to the fast. Since revelations are nearly always received by fasting, this alone will
clarify doctrinal controversial subjects and will prevent
divisions and offences contrary to the true meaning of
the word of God.

Argumentive people who sow discord and divisions
among the followers of Christ are in much need of fasting.
There could be no divisions and very few denominations, if
any at all, if God's people sought Him more through the
prophet's, early church and apostle's length of fasting.
Paul tells us to "MARK THEM" and "AVOID THEM"
that cause divisions because THEY ARE BELLY
SERVERS. This should shame people, who cause friction and sow discord in the church, into fasting. Carnality
becomes so rampant that one cannot see and interpret
truth properly without fastings. Fasting paves the way
for true Holy Ghost prophetical enlightenment of the
word of God. The prophets always found correct and
abundant revelations of the Word of God through fasting. If we want prophecy and unusual experiences we can
have the same experience of the prophets by utilizing
the same secret they used. This is by going into a PROPH-
ET'S—LENGTH FAST.

TWO TWELVE—DAY FASTS:

"My husband and I recently fasted twelve days. The blessings of the Lord just poured thru from Heaven in such a wonderful way.

In my fast, hunger left me the second day, a few days later
I became stronger and felt unusually fine all the way through.

I was surprised at the awful poisons that came out of my
body. We should fast often if it is only to keep ourselves clean.

I wanted to fast longer than twelve days, but we had to move
from our place so I thought I should stop. However, I am going
into a longer one later on. Both my husband and I received such
great Spiritual benefits from these fasts. May God bless you.

Mrs. J. P."
Burbank, Calif.

Another letter from Oron, South Nigeria, West Africa, May 19, 1947, reads in part:

Dear Brother Hall:

I want to tell you that the book "Atomic Power With God" someone sent to me, has come as a direct answer to many of my prayers to God regarding the great revivals He is preparing to send upon us in this part of His vineyard.

I have known the value of a few days of prayer, but lately I have felt a longing for something deeper, but I never knew what it was. Your book proved to be the answer.

How happy I am that I can get so much closer to the Lord in fastings. I previously did not know how to fast more than four days.

I believe the contents of "Atomic Power With God" to be a Heavenly revelation. It has answered many secret questions and many puzzling problems in regard to the Bible.

I have more answers to my prayers and much greater anointing in my life since I have learned how to fast.

Your brother in Christ
J. U. U. (West Africa).

A THIRTEEN-DAY FAST:

Fasting is the answer to many a Christian's needs today. The light on fasting was an answer to my prayer, thank the Lord for it.

I had an awful spiritual warfare when fasting thirteen days. My wife took sick and almost died. Jesus came to our rescue and immediately healed her while I was still on the fast.

I prepared the meals for the rest of my family and my wife.

The first six days I never got more than six or eight hours sleep.

I lost a lot of weight but gained spiritually and physically. I broke the fast because at that time I couldn't seem to pray the way I thought I should. Now I know that it was the old devil trying to get me to doubt. I regret that I didn't go on. As soon as I regain my weight, I intend to go on a twenty-one to forty day fast.

R. A. T.
La Grande, Ore.

Chapter IV

FOOD DRUNKARDS

Medical scientists state that FOOD IS STIMULAT-ING and some kinds of food are more stimulating than others. We agree that it is, and this will explain why our appetites are the product of what we eat. The more stimulating our food, the more our appetites will be stimulated. The more stimulated our appetites become, the more difficult it will be to overcome the FLESHLY NATURE OF THE OLD MAN. The more difficult it is to overcome the flesh, the easier it is for the flesh to overcome the spirit. We should always enjoy the VICTORIOUS, OVER-COMING LIFE, having "been called unto liberty."

If one is to keep the "FLESH CRUCIFIED" as he should, it is advisable not to have a menu that is over-extended with the more stimulating foods. Simplicity in both living and eating will better enable the child of God RETAIN "THE FAITH WHICH WAS ONCE DELIV-ERED UNTO THE SAINTS." If this faith has been lost, fasting and prayer is a method of obtaining it again to the highest degree, along with our consecration.

The over use of even the less stimulating foods will also have stimulating effect upon the body, its cells, and its appetites. The overindulgence in the more stimulating foods will amplify to excess our desire nature and the appetites of the flesh will be more difficult to control. "Walk in the Spirit and ye shall not fulfill the LUST OF THE FLESH." We shall always have to fight for the proper way to live. Proper natural living contributes much towards a better and higher spiritual life of progress for the praise and glory of Jesus Christ. Often the plain and simple teachings of the Scriptures are ignored, and the importance of the Spirit-filled life with the crucifixion of the flesh through food "TEMPERANCE" is not given its proper place. But is it such minor importance?

If food is STIMULATING, the over-use of it will cause "FOOD INTOXICATION" by the "OVERCHARG-

ING" of the cellular tissues. If an individual continues to be "OVERCHARGED WITH SURFEITING," (Luke 21:34), which causes food intoxication, this person becomes a "FOOD DRUNKARD." Food drunkards are everywhere, only they do not conduct themselves in the same manner as alcoholic drunkards do. They suffer physically in the same manner the alcoholic drunkards suffer, but not to the same degree. The strangest thing about it all is that food drunkards seldom realize *surfeiting* is the cause of many of their ills. In fact, most medical experts state that MOST sicknesses and diseases come from the stomach, and can very often be traced to overindulgences in food and drink. This explains why a diagnosis of the condition of the digestional organ is usually made first by way of the tongue. This member is a part of the stomach.

FOOD DRUNKS are those who LIVE TO EAT instead of eating to LIVE. The LIVING TO EAT method insead of eating to live, is what Jesus refers to in Luke 21:34. Jesus also stated, "TAKE HEED (warning) to yourselves, lest at any time your hearts be OVER-CHARGED WITH SURFEITING, and DRUNKEN-NESS, and CARES OF THIS LIFE, so that day come upon you UNAWARES."

Perhaps MOST of the "CARES OF THIS LIFE" concern the problem of food getting or the making of money to purchase it; then follows elaborate over-tasty preparation of it to PLEASE THE APPETITE OF HUN-GER, which in turn feeds the appetites of sex and covetousness. This in turn may lead to temptation and SIN. JESUS CHRIST CONDEMNS THIS, AND TELLS US TO "TAKE HEED". This means WARNING, DANGER LIES AHEAD for those who indulge in it, for the simple reason it may mean the COMING OF THE LORD WILL "COME UPON US UNAWARES."

Satan is very tricky and deceitful, and always uses the method that seems the least harmful to trip God's children. This is most easily done through the pleasure and satisfaction of MAN'S APPETITES.

The story of the race, all down through the ages is nothing more than an account of a series of temptations to satisfy one or more of man's appetites. Eve was tempt-

ed to EAT of the forbidden fruit. She partook of it to
satisfy the lust of the eye and brought the curse of sin
upon the human race. Please do not forget we are continually paying for this sin. Cain became jealous of his
brother Abel and slew him. This was nothing more than
satisfying the appetites of *sex* and *covetous greed.* Esau
let his appetite of HUNGER get out of control. He sold
his birthright to Jacob just to EAT FOOD, and to satisfy
his carnal desire for a few moments of pleasure. In so
doing, he lost everything.

In the days of Noah, "God looked upon the earth,
and, behold, it was corrupt, for all flesh had corrupted his
way upon the earth . . . I will destroy them." Gen. 6:11, 12.
Why? Jesus tells us it was because "THEY WERE EAT-
ING AND DRINKING." Matt. 24:38. It was because
they were satisfying their appetites. Food intoxication was
a contributing cause of the corruption of the flesh to the
extent they had to be destroyed. Fleshly lusts are "contrary" to the Spirit of God. Among many unclean things
caused by them is PRIDE and a self-satisfaction without
God. This is one of the worst abominations in the sight
of God. In the days of Lot it was the same. The appetite
lusts of man were satisfied with pleasure; first it was eating and drinking, and then the SEX lust was stimulated,
followed by all of the corruption that developed to satisfy
these lusts. There was nothing more for God to do except
to send DESTRUCTION because of their uncleanness.

Many have criticized Christ because He condemned
eating along with drinking, but Christ well knew the root
of it all. If there were plenty of fastings and not overindulgences with the food habit, and there could NOT
HAVE BEEN THE INTEMPERANCE OF THE
OTHER APPETITES, because as we have previously
stated, the satisfaction of the appetite of hunger to an
"OVERCHARGED" condition, simply FEEDS THE
OTHER APPETITES. In order to find an outlet for this
over-stimulated condition many seek another form of
pleasure which also could result in sin.

THE ALCOHOL FACTORY

When an excess of carbohydrates, sweets and starches
are eaten, and they go into the stomach to contact the
gastric juices and other acids within, they soon produce

fermentation and form ALCOHOL. Within the body, this alcoholic condition which is caused from certain food excesses and wrong combinations of food, works upon the appetite of hunger in such a manner that it causes HABIT HUNGER. Habit hunger is entirely different from true hunger—the true hunger that returned to Jesus after He had fasted forty days. True real hunger will also return to almost any person fasting around forty days. Habit hunger is the HUNGER LUST for food that causes an individual to become a FOOD DRUNKARD. This alcoholic condition which may be found in Christians as well as sinners, causes them to fall so under the influence of FOOD and EATING as to be unconsciously enslaved in the same manner as alcoholics are bound to the drinking habit. One is the alcoholic habit, and the other is the "habit hunger" eating habit. Both are bound by it. The alcohol generated within the stomach through the over-use of certain foods falsely stimulates the stomach and the appetite of hunger. It whips up this false hunger until one cannot be satisfied with only the amount of food that is needed, and a habit lust is created which is just as bad in God's sight as that for alcohol. We are not free when habit bound.

The Christian tries to fast and finds himself unable to break the food habit because he is bound by it, and about the longest he can go without food is two or three or sometimes four days at a time. This is about the same length of time an alcoholic, or a tobacco fiend can leave off their habits at a time, believe it or not. Yes, many people who wonder why the Lord is not blessing them, may find a solution to this problem right here. I have personally seen hundreds and thousands of individuals go down in repentance and fasting, and find the answers to their PRAYERS.

FOOD DRUNKARDS acquire the habit of over-eating, which is just as much of a habit as the habit of drinking alcohol. It is worse in some respects because the FOOD DRUNKARD is deceived and does not realize he has the habit, while the alcoholic or the drug addict knows he has it. Another way in which it may be worse is that some people, even Christians, have the FOOD HABIT OF SURFEITING nearly all the days of their lives. They die or commit slow suicide many years too soon without knowing they ever had it. Even if they live close enough

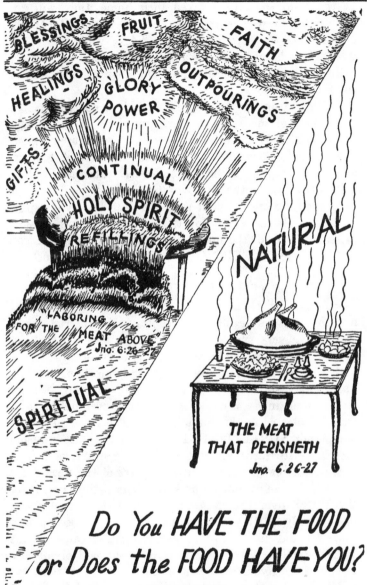

Do You **HAVE THE FOOD**
or Does the **FOOD HAVE YOU?**

Phil. 3:18,19

The Church, today, is shorn of her gifts and power. When the early Church had these, they also put into practice the prophet's length fasts. When this part of the "FAITH" is reinstated within the Church, we again will see the works of the Holy Spirit. The continued stuffing habit, without fasting, will destroy faith and weaken our spirituality. (Matt. 24:38) Can you lay aside food for ten days?

to the Lord to make Heaven their home, they will not
be worthy to receive the CROWN INCORRUPTIBLE.
1 Cor. 9:25. A ten-day or longer FAST will remove the
over-eating habit, and a resumption of careful and proper
eating afterwards will safeguard one against these sins in
the future.

The reason the average layman does not realize the
seriousness of these fleshly lusts, especially of the hunger
lust which feeds the others, is because too many religious
leaders seldom preach a sermon on this kind of temperance, and they never hear the WORD concerning THIS
TRUTH. This is the Word of God, and if you study it
very carefully and without prejudice, and keep your spirit
in tune with the Holy Spirit, I believe you will be surprised to learn of the many beautiful experiences you can
have, just by "KEEPING UNDER" the fleshly lusts of
the OLD MAN. "Feed me with food CONVENIENT FOR
ME: lest I be full, and DENY THEE." (PROV. 30:8, 9.)

Jesus Christ knew a man who *fasted often* and led
a plain and simple life in every way. He ate right, and
had only a very simple menu, in fact, it was the simplest
of fare; most of his life he partook only of two-course meals,
and his appetites were always under subjection. He had
no fleshly lusts or pride with which to contend, because
of his simple mode of living. Many other splendid qualities
were manifested in this humble man, all because he would
not permit SURFEITING. He realized the over-indulged
food appetite feeds all of the other appetites, and it is
a cause for many errors and weaknesses of the flesh. This
wonderful man whom Jesus knew, was living the life of
VICTORY over the *flesh*. Our Lord Jesus Christ spoke
more highly of this man, and gave more praise to him
than He did to any other person, just because of his
VICTORIOUS WAY OF LIVING. Jesus said of him, "I
solemnly tell you that among all of woman born no
GREATER HAS EVER BEEN RAISED UP THAN
JOHN THE BAPTIST." Matt. 11:11. (Weymouth's)

There are too many people who have their eyes on
the natural rather than the spiritual. Jesus said in His
sermon on the mount, "Is not the LIFE more than meat,
and the body than raiment?" Matt. 6:25. In this chapter
Jesus spoke mostly about three major principles, which
were called by the early Christians, the three GREAT

FOUNDATIONS. In them we do homage to our God. They are:

(1.) Alms

(2.) Prayer (the Lord's Prayer)

(3.) Fasting, (and abstemious living)

These are THREE GREAT DUTIES THAT ALL CHRISTIANS SHOULD PRACTICE.

There are four verses in the sixth chapter of Matthew that concern "ALMS." About ten verses have to do with the Lord's Prayer, and there are approximately twelve verses that deal with FASTING and EATING. In other words, more is said upon the subject of fasting and eating than upon any other subject discussed in the sermon on the mount. Nearly every one knows the Lord's prayer, but how many people know about FASTING and temperate LIVING? How many know how to take a prophet's length fast? How many put first things first and second things second and third things third? Yes, we leave off almost entirely the precious powerful truth of fasting. These are God's three great foundations.

"Seek ye *first* the kingdom of God, and His righteousness; and all these things shall be added unto you." Matt. 6:33. Churches minus the third foundation, are tottering

Almsgiving, Prayer, and FASTING are three fundamental processes by which the children of God work out their righteousness after conversion. The average church consistently puts into practice only the first two because they are easier on the flesh than FASTING. To have a balanced SPIRITUAL MEAL, LET US EAT THE WHOLE WORD OF GOD!

STIMULATING EATABLES

Since we have seen that food acts as a stimulant in the way and manner it CHARGES our two million cells, it might be well to study just how much stimulating quality food has in it. The less stimulating the food is, the easier it is to keep down the lusts of the flesh. There is less of a tendency toward overindulgence in the partaking of the less stimulating foods. Undernourished individuals who are suffering from malnutrition are not asked to consider this chart too much. The purpose of the chart is to aid the great majority of persons who find it difficult to keep the body under, and the flesh subdued. I present it only so

it will be a spiritual blessing, and to show how important
is the part food plays in our lives in keeping down the old
man. The left side of the chart shows the food that is
less stimulating, and it increases from left to right.

When on a FAST the individual is free from all the
stimulating influences that food gives, except for the first
few days of the fast. It usually requires at least four days,
or even more, before certain bulk food materials are
broken down, and the residue removed. This may be true
to some extent even when enemas are taken. The stimulation at this time is very low, and while some food particles, food rust, corrosion, and contaminated morbid material may remain in the intestinal tract for more than a
month, the stimulation in the fast will remain at about
ZERO after the first few days.

The longer FOOD ABSTENTION continues, the more
complete becomes this housecleaning process in the intestinal tract, and in the two million vital cells of the human
electric plant. This is why a longer fast than just several
days is much more efficient in enabling one to reach out
for great spiritual things.

The STIMULATING character of food is natural and
gives to one in health a feeling of energy, pep, pleasure,
and well-being. When food abstention begins, the whole
being goes into a period of acclimation. As the participant
keeps himself in consecration, a transition from the natural
to the spiritual occurs. As there are no stimulating influences to continue to whip up the NATURAL, and much
of this may be likened unto a puffed up balloon, the
spiritual will be more easily within his reach. One does
not have the capacity to enjoy even the simple natural
pleasures of every day life. This is another reason fasting
seems so difficult. Fasting lays aside these stimulating influences which the natural man must have in order to
have pleasure. This denial of self opens up to us a NEW
APPETITE for another kind of menu that is also STIMU-
LATING, only it is the STIMULATING influence of the
SPIRIT, and the MENU will be FEAST ON HEAVENLY
MANNA AND THE GREAT GLORIES OF GOD.
Much of the Word of God will be revealed to us in a great
new spiritual light and understanding. We will have power
to get under the great burden for others. Greater things
will be done through us so others can have a blessing,

(STIMULATING POWER)

AIR ●
WATER ●

FASTING

(NON-STIMULATING)

VEGETABLE JUICES (raw)

Group No. 1

- Fruit juices
- Fresh Citrus fruits
- Sour or buttermilk
- Raw eggs
- Milk and sweet fruit
- Green vegetables
- Salad
- Thin soup
- Soups and Vegetables
- Lentiles
- Honey
- Peas
- Heavy cooked vegetables
- Whole cereals Grain
- (Locusts) Puddings Gravies

Group No. 2

- Fried foods
- Meats roasts
- Fish and Stewed chicken
- Smoked meats
- Heavy pastries
- Candy Fried meats
- Baked beans
- (Fats) Red meats

Group No. 3

- Coffee
- Tea
- Certain sauces Pickles Chili Tamales
- Beer and Light alcoholic drinks
- Pepper Condiments (Spices)
- Sweet wines
- Tobacco
- Sour wines
- Dope Narcotics Drugs
- Whiskey Liquor

(Non-eatables)

CHART depicting the stimulating character of foods. The latter stimulants may not be classified as food, but are included for comparison and should be classified as non-eatables. WATER IS NOT FOOD, THEREFORE IT IS NOT STIMULATING and is taken when fasting. All food whips up and feeds carnality. The more stimulating food is, the greater carnality.

whether it is a burden for the unsaved or for a fellow Christian brother or sister. A spiritual gift may also be received when earnestly sought.

WATER DRINKING NOT STIMULATING

Food and drink (beverage) are two entirely different things. Fasting means to do without food entirely and does not exclude the use of pure water, which is a type of the blessed Holy Spirit, and of Salvation. The "drink" in olden times also included poisonous beverages like the alcoholic and drug drinks of today. WATER IS IN NO WAY STIMULATING TO THE BODY OR TO THE APPETITES. It aids in neutralizing the stimulating tendencies of the food, and an individual becomes "undone" far quicker by the drinking of water than by doing without it. If the stimulating power of water is zero, then it stands to reason water drinking in the fast will greatly aid the candidate in the subjugation of the natural appetites. Drink does not always mean water in the Bible.

So far as the health is concerned, short fasts without water are immaterial, but it is absolutely necessary to drink water while on the "complete fast." This is a fast from the time hunger leaves until hunger returns. On any fast which continues for more than a few days, the drinking of water is essential. If an individual takes a forty-day fast and is under the power the entire time, or is in the power of God as Moses was, he can go on this "HUNGER AND THIRST." (II Cor. 11:27) for the entire time without water and without harm. Very likely there will be many other things one can do in this state that they can not do outside of the supernatural powers of God. This is exceptional, however. We are dealing with the fast any individual can take to glorify Jesus Christ, and receive wonderful physical results as well as spiritual. After all, the first step to Godliness is cleanness of the body.

Even when an individual goes on a hunger and a thirst fast without drinking water, does he actually do without water entirely? I say he is getting some water anyway, whether he drinks it or not. He is getting it through his skin and through the air he breathes. The more dense the air is, the more water is absorbed into his body in this manner.

Dr. J. H. Kellogg, of the Battle Creek Sanitarium,

says: "From the skin which is abundantly supplied with lymph vessels, water and many substances in solution may be absorbed, and thus taken into the system. A case is on record in which a boy in London Hospital suffering with diabetes, absorbed nine pints of fluid through the skin in twenty-four hours."

Dr. Luduc has shown conclusively that certain drugs can be introduced into the tissues via the skin.

Professor Kahlenber says: "It is remarkable that in five minutes after the feet are immersed in the boric acid solution, boric acid is present in the urine."

If these facts are true how can a person go in a fast without getting water into his system and obey the directions of Jesus Christ in dedicating and consecrating the fast to Him? In Matthew 6:17: "But thou, when thou fastest, anoint thine head, and *WASH THY FACE;*" We should anoint ourself with oil which is the type of the Holy Spirit, or we can be anointed by the elders of the church and set apart for the fast. The anointing makes the fast more sacred and it is more consecrated. It will help enable us to more successfully complete the dedicated fast. The washing of our face is also a sign of cleanliness and makes us inconspicious. When we wash and bathe, our system will of course absorb water. If the diabetic absorbed over a gallon of water into his system through his skin, naturally a person that "washes himself" will also absorb water, so how can a person do entirely without water?

FAST: Abstinence from food; religious MORTIFICATION (Col. 3:5) by abstinence. (Webster)

FOOD: Nourishment of nutriment.

NOURISHMENT: Food.

THIRST: A sensation of dryness in the throat, mouth, and stomach; a great desire to drink.

Christ did not thirst after His forty day fast, He HUNGERED.

For instance, water is designated "H_2O" (H for hydrogen, and O for oxygen). It is two parts hydrogen and one part oxygen. The atomic combining weight of hydrogen is 1; the combining weight of oxygen is 16. Then to 18 pounds of water, God carefully measures out 2 pounds of hydrogen and 16 pounds of oxygen from the air we breathe. Water can be formed only by mixing these gases together and in these exact proportions. Since the air is full of moisture (small particles of water), no individual can fast without water entirely whether he realizes it or not. The nostrils and skin breathes small particles of moisture into the body.

The two elements of water and air are the non-stimulants that can get into our stomach and not cause "FOOD DRUNKENNESS." From these non-stimulants we can trace the stimulating power of food right up to the class of foods in group three, which are the non-eatable group, that is, they are from the group we should not eat or drink. These are far more stimulating than the food found in groups one and two. Some of the foods found in group one are "pulse foods" which Daniel and his comrades chose to eat, rather than the more stimulating food found in group three which was called the "portion of the King's meat." Dan. 1:13. This is the group which may be called "no pleasant bread." Dan. 10:3. The appetites are not stimulated nearly as much with these foods as with those found in the other groups. One can get closer to the Spirit realm on a diet of the foods in this group rather than on a diet of the foods in the last two groups. However, dieting does not take the place of fasting. Food abstention is still a step closer to the spiritual than light dieting. I do not expect an individual to follow indefinitely as light a diet as may be found in group one; I point out only the lesser stimulating foods which can be used when an individual wishes to seek God more effectively, and yet not go on the fast. The fast, of course, will be the most effective spiritual method of obtaining the ATOMIC POWER WITH GOD.

THE TOBACCO, ALCOHOLIC, AND DOPE HABIT CURE

The FOOD INTOXICATION HABIT has about the same grip on the average individual as the habit of tobacco or alcohol, believe it or not! Food is stimulating and so is alcohol, only alcohol reaches the blood stream quicker, penetrates faster, and has a far greater degree of stimulating qualities. Alcohol is the stronger stimulant, but both stimulate and whip up the appetites of *hunger, sex, and covetous greed.* Try for a period of thirty days to eat half or two thirds the quantity of food you have been accustomed to eating, and note how difficult it is to do this. It is about as difficult to do this as it is for the alcoholic or cigarette fiend to try to cut down by one half the habits of drinking or smoking. If you are not accustomed to fasting, just observe how hard it is to continue food abstention for only ten days. It is just as difficult to do without God's help, as it is for a person to break the alcohol or tobacco habit. Usually many attempts are made, and much effort is expended before either habit is conquered. The same thing applies to the starting of a consecration fast, and to its continuance for ten days or longer.

The comparison just made, may seem shocking to some individuals, but should it be? Even the child of God at times is bound unknowingly by the food habit, and is a slave to the "EATABLES" of which God said, "In sorrow shalt thou eat of it all the days of thy life." If one has never taken a fast of any length, it is easy to say he does not believe it, but let him go on a hunger strike for ten days, and see for himself.

When food abstention begins, the elimination of the sorrow that is connected with the food also begins. One no longer is eating of something under the curse but is opening up new channels through which the Holy Spirit can **FEED US WITH THE HEAVENLY MANNA.** Go on a hunger strike and strike out the devil for a season; let your appetites have a holiday.

Is it any wonder then, that God does not always answer the prayers of very precious souls? Many times the individual does pray earnestly and fervently. and God gives him the desire of his heart. God looks upon his heart and excuses his ignorance concerning some of his habits of living because he has not yet learned the better way.

Most habits that are the result of certain cravings from the stomach, such as hunger, smoking, drinking, dope, and the use of narcotics, *have their roots centered in the heart of the stomach.* There is the smoking hunger, the drinking hunger, the dope hunger, and the food hunger, as well as many others which can be separated, but still have their deep roots in the **MASTER HUNGER APPETITE.** The one appetite of hunger holds the key to all lesser habits along this line. The key to control the main appetite of hunger is nothing more than **FOOD ABSTENTION.** Abstention from food goes right to the source of all of these habits. Atlhough they might have been of long standing and very acute, including morphine, marijuana, and other deadly drugs, these roots can be unfastened and eradicated through FASTING. Usually a two week fast will be sufficient, but sometimes it may require longer. A twenty-one day fast will easily get rid of any habit, though it usually is not necessary to fast more than two weeks. After the fast, there will be no more desire for any of these habits unless the person himself re-instates the craving for them. There will be a new habit acquired in regard to proper eating if the candidate will use discretion in the manner in which his fast is broken.

When a person tries to break the alcoholic or drug habit, and continues eating, even though he shall abstain from it for ten or fifteen days, food continues to feed the roots of it. This just fans it so the evil craving is not eradicated completely, and it will very likely return at some other time and its practice be continued. Fasting is the sure method for correction of any of these habits, and is the quickest cure. The habit itself is actually consumed in the fast.

Here is the testimony of a Christian brother who had tried every means to free himself from the cigarette habit, until he heard about the FASTING WAY:

> "I fasted two weeks without food and I praise Jesus for delivering me of the cigarette habit.
>
> "After three days of fasting, hunger left me, and the desire for smoking left entirely. Toward the end of the fast when I bathed daily, the water was coated with the brownish color of nicotine. Fasting so loosened up the desire the old roots and even the old poisons came right out of my system, and I have had no further desire for it. The fast so cleaned me up in fourteen days the Lord baptized me in the Holy Spirit. I was twenty-nine pounds underweight before fasting. I gained not only the sixteen pounds back that I lost while fasting but I gained twenty-nine more pounds. Sixty days later I weighed exactly what I was supposed to weigh. All nervousness, sleeplessness, and stomach trouble entirely diappeared. I feel better than I have felt in twenty years, thank my Saviour."
>
> Charles Wilson, San Diego, Calif.

Attention is now called to the fact that some foods stimulate the natural appetites more than foods of lesser stimulating effects. Alcohol and certain drugs are far more stimulating than food, but they operate in the same manner as food, except they are amplified many times in their stimulating characteristics. A person under the influence of alcohol will have a much stronger sex desire, and weaker moral sensibilities than when not under this influence. The same is true when one is under the influence of dope, tobacco poisoning, or even much heavy stimulating food.

It is man's appetites that cause him either to sin, or to accomplish some noble worthy purpose, such as reproduction in holy matrimony; or the covetous appetite will give him a normal desire to care for the family and render good service at his job, or in his business. A proper covetous desire is good.

A fast sanctifies and makes dormant these appetites for the time, and one is more able to reach God in this state than in any other. After fasting they return in a normal sanctified manner. To show how alcohol or any other strong stimulant operates on the appetites, one may observe that a person under the influence of liquor may have a greater appetite to eat; the appetite of hunger may be stimulated, not only for more food but for more drink as well. A partially drunken man may steal a fine automobile which he had wanted when sober. With highly stimulating alcohol or drugs whipping up the covetous appetite, he chooses to yield to the temptation of obtaining it by a method which is both morally wrong and criminal.

Food also works on the appetites but to a lesser degree. Fasting places them at zero so far as stimulation is concerned, and the evidence presented points to the fact that THE FASTING PRAYER is very necessary in the Christian's life.

FASTING OR FEASTING

The natural man likes to FEAST, the consecrated child of God loves to go on FASTS. Which shall it be, FASTING OR FEASTING? To me there is very little difference in these words, but to the carnal person there is a wide difference. There should not be much difference between FASTING and FEASTING to the Christian!

After all if the "E" was taken out of FEASTING we would have FASTING. Even without changing the word, "FEASTING," it should not make a lot of difference to Holy Spirit filled people, because when we go into FAST-INGS, we still are in FEASTINGS. This time the menu has been changed from the natural food to the MANNA from ABOVE. It is the FEAST OF GREAT SPIRITUAL THINGS. Let us go on a FAST, and enjoy some of the wonderful FEASTING experiences to be had from GOD. *Give your stomach a vacation and let your belly have a holiday.*

It is difficult to be engaged in two major interests at one time and make a success of both. This applies also to spiritual things. If we want to reach real heights, and to become a great blessing to others, it is necessary to sur-render the natural, the fleshly, the earthly, the appetites, and everything else, to God. Then we are on the road to winning victories, which have never been won. This is the FASTING-FEASTING ROAD of food abstention. It is an unpopular road, but the few there be who have ex-perienced it have tasted things no other person has tasted. PAUL experienced it often, and some of his experiences were so rich, and sacred, he was forbidden to utter them.

The FASTING-FEASTING experience requires the abolition of the three natural appetites (temporarily). Food abstention is the only process known which will accomplish this. These natural appetites must be starved out of the way, and FASTING guarantees that this will be done. It is sin that seeks to use them as a strong hold from which to work effectively. They become dormant in the fast. They are still there, but they are inoperative for the time being. Please do not misunderstand me, although these appetites are dormant, an individual can still permit sin to come into his being and operate through his flesh, but he does not want to and cannot care too much for them while fasting. The desire nature is not under stimu-lation, consequently a person is under favorable influences toward the spiritual, and if prayer and advancement towards this goal is made, the person is susceptible to high spiritual influences. There is a great temptation during the first part of the fast, to yield to the appetite of hun-ger. This is also the key to the other appetites of SEX and the COVETOUS NATURE. Hereunder are catalogued some of the works or lusts of the flesh which pertain to man's three natural appetites.

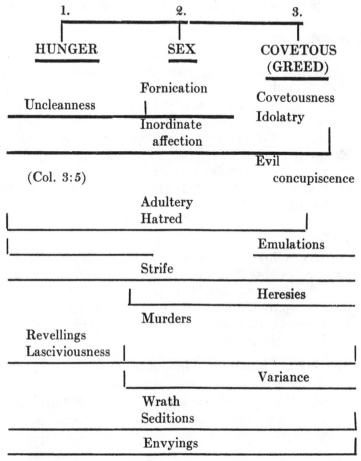

Drunkeness

Witchcraft is traced to the abnormal lower side of the spiritual appetite. (Galatians 5:19-21.)

The works of the flesh are shown as they tend to lean in the direction of the appetites. Some are related to more than one of the appetites. In FASTINGS, the appetites are so dormant these fleshly lusts cannot operate to the same extent they could when not fasting. The varying power of the different works of the flesh will not all be cut down in the same proportion. Some will be almost nil, while others may be retarded only slightly. Then too, during the first part of the fast, while the heavy poisons are loosening up, some could be even worse than they would be when eating. For example, generally speaking, people are very cross and easily provoked to anger when the stomach is empty. If several meals have been missed, their condition seems to become worse, for the simple reason the quality of fuel the energies are consuming at that time is very poor. In the beginning of food abstention there is the old polluted, worn down, rotten, vile material, and fecal matter from which blood is continually being saturated with poisons. This is brought through most of the body in the process of elimination and cleansing, and naturally these appetites and fleshly lusts are going to feel certain effects from it, and the worst side of them all is brought out. It requires days for the temple of the Holy Spirit to become clean before the full display of the mastery and "MORTIFICATION" of the "MEMBERS" takes place.

The "OLD MAN" is a very hard foe to conquer. He has been pampered, caressed, and fed so much with things that PLEASE the flesh, it is only with a great struggle he gives up. Col. 3:9, 10. The prophets and apostles knew these secrets, that is why the prophet's length fast will master the situation.

LONG FAST RENEWED BODY AND SOUL

A gentleman fasted thirty-one days at the age of seventy, now he is eighty-four and writes this testimony:

"I am glad for what fasting has done for me. At seventy I took my longest fast, thirty-one days. Although I have fasted many times for two and three weeks without food, only water taken, I began to be depressed in spirit, and wanted to take a long fast. I started out fasting in a very weakened condition physically, but had a glorious renewing of my whole body, soul, and spirit. I came out of the fast with a new liver, a new stomach, new kidneys, a new body. Every cell in my body was cleansed. I am eighty-four now and believe the fasts helped me to live longer. I am thankful for all that the Lord has done for me."

S. M. S.

Lincoln, Neb.

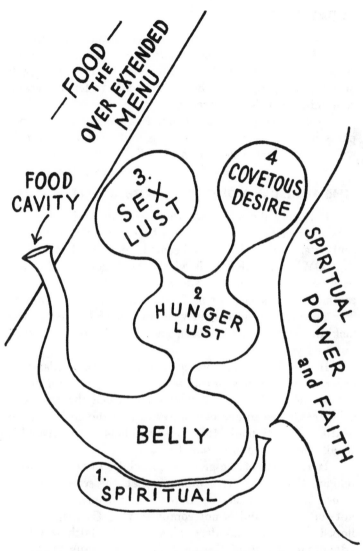

THE FOOD BABIES
THE FOUR APPETITES
Depicting the surfeiter (Luke 21:34).

95% of the American people are auto-intoxicated from an overcharged food condition (surfeiting), state medical authorities. Food drunkards are everywhere. The continued stuffing habit kills more faith and more Spirit than most other evils. "His natural face in a glass."

13 DAY FAST

"I have had severe stomach trouble and nervousness. After fasting and praying for thirteen days, and with criticism, I decided to break the fast. After a few days of eating properly, I feel better than I have felt for years. A number of things cleared up.

"I only regret that I did not fast longer. I had some pains in my muscles while fasting, but now I know this was a normal condition of the fast."

Mr. F. G. E., Portland, Oregon

THE TREASURE HOUSE OF SPIRITUAL EXPERIENCES

It is very doubtful that the Christian world ever will fully appreciate a truth that has been concealed for many centuries. Although it has been "hidden in plain sight," the POWER THEREOF is within the finger tips of us all, because Jesus not only made no secret of the way of attainment, but also gave us THE KEY in explicit words. The door has been in plain view and the KEY left in the lock, but somehow it has been passed by for over nineteen hundred years.

In the Agronchoda Parechai verses of the Vedas it is ordered that seventy priests over seventy years old guard the law of the Lotus, that whoever revealed the secrets of a higher degree to one of a lower degree should be put to death. JESUS made this very precious truth available to all; there is no premium to pay.

Here is one of the greatest principles of the Christian religion that is far more valuable than the secrets as contained in the law of the Lotus and the priests. This is not for sinners and is not compulsory to Christians. It is hoped, however, that deep pillars of the faith will take advantage of one of the most effective means known to man of obtaining a treasure house of SPIRITUAL RICHES AND GLORY. We would like to induce every reader to TAKE HOLD OF THE KEY, ENTER THE DOOR, AND RECEIVE THE GIFTS OF THE SPIRIT, as well as many surprises lying in store for him.

FASTING AND PRAYER MEANS MUCH IN HAWAII

"Dear Brother Hall:

Your book on Fasting and Prayer came to me through a Filipino Brother. I feel it is the message for the hour.

I want to distribute the books; please find enclosed order for some.

Fasting means much in our labors for Him out here. We hope to get the truth out more and more so greater revivals will begin.

H. S."
Haikee, Main
T. H.   (Hawaii)

The author has sent many books and tracts to Honolulu. The fasting "contagion" is spreading in that area too. Many are fasting ten days and longer. We hear reports that the Lord is blessing in healings and souls are being converted. Praise His name forever.

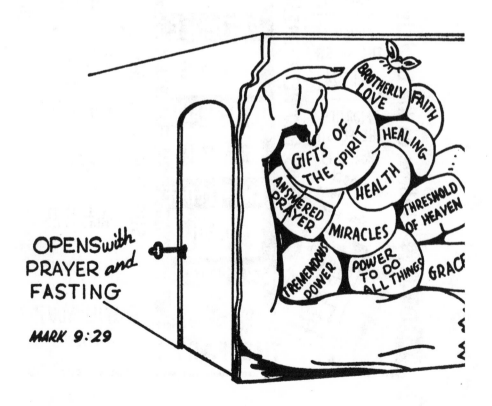

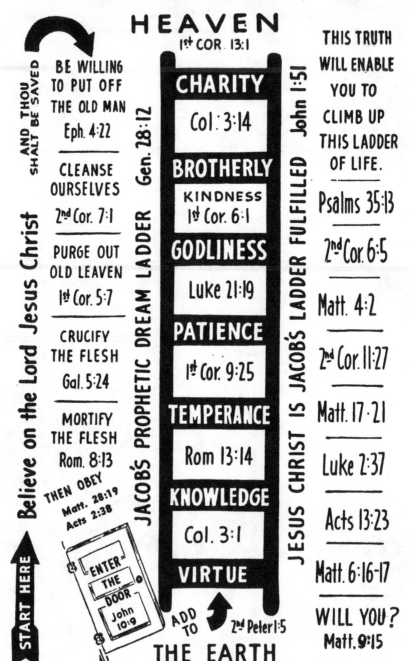

THE WAY OF LIFE
ST. JOHN 14:6

HEAVEN
1st COR. 13:1

AND THOU SHALT BE SAVED

BE WILLING TO PUT OFF THE OLD MAN
Eph. 4:22

CLEANSE OURSELVES
2nd Cor. 7:1

PURGE OUT OLD LEAVEN
1st Cor. 5:7

CRUCIFY THE FLESH
Gal. 5:24

MORTIFY THE FLESH
Rom. 8:13

THEN OBEY
Matt. 28:19
Acts 2:38

Believe on the Lord Jesus Christ

START HERE

JACOB'S PROPHETIC DREAM LADDER
Gen. 28:12

CHARITY
Col. 3:14

BROTHERLY
KINDNESS
1st Cor. 6:1

GODLINESS
Luke 21:19

PATIENCE
1st Cor. 9:25

TEMPERANCE
Rom 13:14

KNOWLEDGE
Col. 3:1

VIRTUE

ADD TO
2nd Peter 1:5

ENTER THE DOOR
John 10:9

THE EARTH

John 1:51

JESUS CHRIST IS JACOB'S LADDER FULFILLED

THIS TRUTH WILL ENABLE YOU TO CLIMB UP THIS LADDER OF LIFE.

Psalms 35:13

2nd Cor. 6:5

Matt. 4:2

2nd Cor. 11:27

Matt. 17:21

Luke 2:37

Acts 13:23

Matt. 6:16-17

WILL YOU?
Matt. 9:15

Chart used thru the courtesy of Azusa News, Box 4907, Los Angeles 1, Calif.

Chapter V

DANIEL'S DIET AND FASTS

Daniel 1:8-20: "Daniel purposed in his heart that he would not defile himself with the portion of the king's meat, nor with the wine which he drank: therefore he requested of the prince of the eunuchs that he might NOT DEFILE HIMSELF. Now God had brought Daniel into favour and tender love with the prince of the eunuchs.

" (10) And the prince of the eunuchs said unto Daniel, I fear my lord the king, who hath appointed your meat and your drink: for WHY SHOULD HE SEE YOUR FACES WORSE LIKING THAN THE CHILDREN WHICH ARE YOUR SORT? then shall ye make me endanger my head to the king. (11) Then said Daniel to Melzar, whom the prince of the eunuchs had set over Daniel, Hananiah, Mishael, and Azariah, (12) Prove thy servants, I beseech thee, ten days; and let them give us pulse (vegetable like) to eat, and water to drink. (13) Then let our countenances be looked upon before thee, and the countenance of the children that eat of the portion of the king's meat: and as thou seest, deal with thy servants. (14) So he consented to them in this matter, and proved them ten days. (15) At the end of ten days their countenance appeared fairer and fatter in flesh than all the children which did eat the portion of the king's meat.

" (17) As for these four children, God gave them knowledge and skill in all learning and wisdom: and Daniel had understanding IN ALL VISIONS AND DREAMS. (18) . . . the prince of the eunuchs brought them in before Nebuchadnezzar. (19) And the king communed with them; and *among them all was found none like Daniel, Hananiah, Mishael,* and *Azariah*: therefore stood they before the king. (20) And in all matters of wisdom and understanding, that the king enquired of them, he found them ten times better than all the magicians and astrologers that were in all his realm."

The book of Daniel is a product of FASTING AND

PRAYER. It consists of one dream and four visions of revelations. Daniel was no more entitled to these revelations than any other Jew, but since he had sought God with an undefiled diet and by prayer and fasting, it was given to him. Daniel was honored to have the revelations for his people.

The message contained in the first chapter of Daniel is very fitting for a person seeking after God's own heart in order that he may be emptied of the sensual appetites of the natural to be able to receive the spiritual.

Several things are noted about Daniel in this chapter:

(1.) He was familiar with the right and wrong ways of living. Daniel put God first.

(2.) He was a dietarian, and he abstained from the food that would prevent God's blessing from resting upon him to the fullest extent. He knew what to eat that was beneficial to health, and what type of diet would insure the continued presence of God in his life. He led an abstemious life. In other words, what is good for the natural man is also good for the spiritual. Harm to the body is likewise harm to the spiritual nature. Daniel followed a simplified menu rather than an over-extended one.

(3.) In this instance, Daniel was a vegetarian. The pulse that was eaten was vegetables. It is far easier to receive revelations from the spirit realm when eating vegetables, or eating nothing at all, than when eating heavy food and meat.

(4.) Daniel would not under any consideration defile himself by over-indulgence, let alone by eating the heavy food from the king's table, even if it should cost the life of his friend, the eunuch, Verse 10.

(5.) Daniel took care of his physical body.

(6.) Daniel was acquainted with "FASTING" and dieting. He was not in ignorance like the world of his day. He had practiced food temperance and fasting to the extent that he knew the value of the process. In Daniel's day, as today, the average person felt that

he had to be on a three or four meal a day
eating schedule in order to "appear" good,
feel well, and not hasten toward the grave.
Daniel astounded everyone after the ten-
day test.

(7.) Daniel's diet made him appear "FAT-
TER AND FAIRER" than the children of
the world.

(8.) Consequently, "Daniel had *understanding* in all *visions* and *dreams*."

(9.) Daniel and his comrades were ten times
better than all the magicians and astrologers
that were in the king's realm.

(10.) Daniel knew God through prayer and
fasting and was prayed up.

The results of this ten-day *test* of proper eating not
only gave Daniel and his companions high favor with the
king by breaking down certain false ideas and prejudices
concerning the lust for food, but it went a long way in
giving Daniel high favor with his God, and in establishing
a sound foundation for the higher blessings from the
Lord of heaven that were to be his later on. How fitting
this should be in the first chapter. His experience should
be a great lesson to the American people today.

THE SOAP PLANT

In America, during and after the second world war,
we heard much said about "waste." "Save fats," for soaps.
Ammunition, soaps and soap powders are made from fats
and have become very scarce. The excess fats some
individuals eat in a day, would make enough soap to do
an average family's weekly washing.

Not only is there an excess of fat in the average
person's stomach, but that very stomach is converted into
a "SOAP" manufacturing plant when an insufficient
amount of bile is available to digest and aid in the ab-
sorption of the fats. The fats go into soap and may clog
the bile ducts. When there is little or no bile in the intestines, tests have shown that anywhere from 22 percent
to 58 percent of the fat intake is found in the feces practically undigested, and in a soapy condition. Sometimes
a person will belch up this fatty soap-like substance, or
take magnesia, bromo seltzer, aspirin, or something of the

kind, which all points to an admission of his guilt and
SIN. You might ask yourself these questions: IS my
body a SOAP PLANT? Can I expect the Holy Spirit to
keep me anointed when He has to occupy a soap plant?

Daniel WOULD NOT BE GUILTY OF SUCH DE-
FILEMENT, therefore we have the reason why God
could use Daniel.

Any Christian can make this simple test. Eat light
foods for ten days and see how much more beautiful your
complexion becomes. Note how much more easily you
can pray when the stomach is in a comfortable, uncrowded
condition than when you have an overloaded stomach.
It is also easier for a sinner to seek the Lord while eating
vegetables rather than heavy food and meat dishes.

In dealing with the subject of light eating and fasting, please do not be misled into fasting or dieting lightly
if you are undernourished and already half starved. Some
folk try fasting, eating unbalanced light diets, or go on a
menu that is so deficient in the minerals and vitamins
their bodies need that they break down and suffer much
physically.

Our body is like a storage battery. When a battery
goes down, it will not have any more energy until it is
recharged. Likewise when we have fasted a large number
of days we should be fully rested and recuperated before
fasting again. The same thing applies to light eating and
full eating. It takes a very long time to become fully
recuperated from a long fast of three weeks or more. In
other words, let us use common sense and not overdo a
good thing. I am adding this caution here because some
folk become so delighted when they find out about this
new source of power with God that they tend to become
over-zealous, to their physical hurt.

Some claim they can go on a very light diet, and have
splendid results with God. This may be true, but unless
you know the type of diet on which to go for your own
minimum daily requirements, you may find one harmful
if long drawn out. It is less harmful in most cases to go
on an absolute fast than on a light diet for the simple
reason the physiological process is very natural when fasting, and the waste and body fats supply in the right
amounts the elements that are necessary for the normal
functions of the body; while on a light diet, you may be

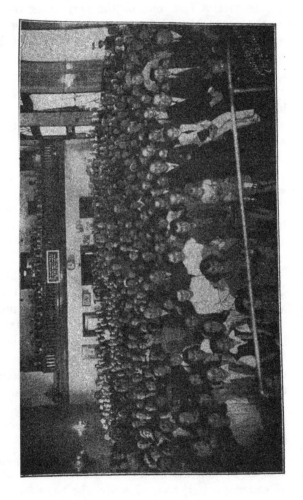

All nation's revival campaign, June 20, 1947, Halstead Spanish auditorium (Chicago, Ill.). Hundreds were converted and scores started fasting for the old time faith and the gifts of the Spirit. (Our group on a fast).

supplying the right amounts of some things to the body but may be failing to supply it with others. While the certain things are only partly supplied, the body will be breaking down from the work it is doing in caring for the assimilative and eliminative work of what is given it to do, and the strain from that which is lacking will deteriorate and unbalance the entire system.

In fact, a fast may be the very thing that is needed in the natural, to bring a person to feeling better. In other words, sick people may become well by fasting. Many thin people are thin because their functional glands and organs are so burdened and overworked from food over-indulgence they cannot take on weight no matter how much they eat. I have seen many thin and underweight people gain weight and become of normal weight after a fast of ten days or more followed by weeks of careful eating. In many instances all that was wrong was that they needed to give their organs a much needed vacation and their belly a holiday.

Man is the shortest lived creature on earth. If he lived eight times his growth period, as is the case with animals, he would have an average life span of one hundred ninety-two years. Instead, he matures at about twenty-one, and does well to reach an average age of fifty-six years.

Man drinks the same water, breathes the same air and lives under the same sunshine as do animals. The great difference between them and the contrast in their life span is in their food. Man eats too much, and eats too many things. He eats too often. When he eats too much he creates a terrific burden for his digestive apparatus. When he eats too many things a chemical inharmony, or what we call indigestion, is set up. If he eats fewer foods, but in bad combinations, it causes fermentation and irritation.

And so it goes. Instead of using his intelligence, man acts as though his head were made for the sole purpose of wearing a hat; and, of course, he pays for his indiscretions with suffering, pain and discomfort as well as a great loss of spiritual power, and the distance between him and his God becomes greater.

Daniel very well knew the significance of proper and improper eating and had wisdom in certain spiritual values as well. He counted it most important to live a life of plainness and simplicity so he could be always in the proper relationship with his God. He was always on talking terms, so to speak, with the Lord. No kind of food would be permitted to dull that focusing point of heavenly contact.

Unless one is performing heavy manual labor, two meals a day when properly selected and combined give ample nourishment. In some cases one meal is sufficient. The older a person becomes the less food he requires.

The three-meal-a-day system was adopted many years ago to meet the requirement of man when he produced his own food by heavy muscular exertion . . . that is to say, when agriculture was his chief pursuit. Three meals a day, especially in the summer, unless they are light and well spaced, will give us more nourishment than we need. A man doing heavy work breathes deeply and burns the food he eats to harmless forms. He may require more food than those performing lighter work.

We are now in the aquarian age, the era of the machine, and no longer can utilize properly great quantities of food. The machine is now doing most of man's work.

If it was necessary for Daniel and his companions to eat sparingly in their day when there was no modern machinery, is it not much more important for man to have a simple diet and to FAST to his God in this day with all of it's labor saving devices.

Let us learn about food and fasting from Daniel.

Both cancer and diabetes are on the increase. Surely if people knew that by right living with *fasting* these two dreadful diseases could be warded off and prevented, they would do something about it.

The Cancer Society states that "cancer spreads throughout the body and is fatal." Yet they say "it is not a blood disease." There is only one way that it can spread throughout the body, and that is through the bloodstream. Therefore, the cancer must be a part of this vital fluid. When the circulatory processes have deposited the cancer cells in certain parts of the body, and the growth is removed by surgery, what becomes of the cancer poisons which the blood has deposited previous to the operation? We believe this to be a polluted condition of the blood caused by the sin of over-eating and wrong living.

Dr. Northen's experiment with animals and soil

chemistry has given the world much valuable information. An experiment Dr. Northen has made with rats feeding on a diet similar to that of residents of a community in which stomach ulcers are very prevalent caused the rats likewise to have stomach ulcers.

Experiments worked on rats and mice in Chicago definitely prove that the irritating matter coming from canned foods, preservatives, spices, and drugs will produce cancer in the animals eating such foods. By placing the rats and mice on proper nutrition this condition was prevented.

Government reports show one person in eight will die of cancer every year.

If animals get cancer by eating our spiced up, over-seasoned, depleted food, then why should we expect to overcome the consequences of such eating?

Rats fed the diet of the Britisher take on the temperament of the British people. When the Sikh diet is fed rats, they become huge and have soulful eyes, the same as the followers of the Hindu sect.

Mankind is also a product of what he eats. This is true both physically and spiritually.

Fasting will help undo the evil of wrong eating and enable the Christian to be a product of a spiritual menu.

A Johanna Brandt of South Africa, was entirely cured of the awful disease of cancer by fasting many times for ten to twelve days, and then she went on a long grape diet.

In both San Francisco and Chicago, I am personally acquainted with doctors who are putting cancer patients on a twelve to fifteen day fast followed by raw vegetable and fruit juices, and many are cured. Dr. Bergen, a Christian physician in Chicago, tell me of one of his patients who became completely cured of cancer by taking many short fasts and then a long one of eighty-four days.

Fasting is a part of right living; without it one cannot keep the temple of the Holy Spirit clean. It works both spiritually and physically.

If many sicknesses are caused by improper eating, is it any wonder that many people have difficulty in getting healed in healing meetings? If they were healed some of them would go out and over-indulge the food lust again; they would be down in a few weeks by satisfying carnality and be ready to come back again to God for healing of sickness caused by yielding to the appetites. It is God's will to heal, but we must live right afterwards. "Sin no more, lest a worse thing come upon thee." John 5:14.

Christians who are seeking to be healed need to get cleaned up and live right, search themselves, and ask God to reveal to them their trouble. Many times it is easier for sinners to be healed than for Christians. One can never fully realize the importance of the sin of over-indulgence until he takes a fast, then he suddenly awakes. The original sin of the fall of man becomes quickened into sudden realization.

"My people are destroyed for lack of knowledge because thou hast rejected knowledge." Hosea 4:6. Physical destruction as well as spiritual decay is everywhere just because people reject the powerful truth of fasting.

Oh yes, Daniel had as good an appetite as anyone, but he knew how to say no! He would not be "destroyed."

Many of God's people when brought before a lovely dinner with an over extended menu, eat, then over-eat, saying it looks too tempting to pass by, and while they are eating they are remembering their medicine cabinet instead of sanctified consecration. In a few months or years some of these individuals will have broken down somewhere with one or more disorders or growths which any physician knows are caused by auto-intoxication brought on by overeating.

Tumors, cancer, ulcers, indigestion, kidney disorders, gout, palsy, goiter and nervous debility are some of the ailments frequently caused by indulgence in the lust of overeating.

In the last days of this dispensation men will be "LOVERS OF PLEASURES MORE THAN LOVERS OF GOD." Overeating becomes a gross sin when a person lives to eat instead of eating to live.

Let us be like Daniel and try to do our best even in little things, for the Glory of God. Let us deny ourselves carnal pleasure for Godly pleasures.

This was Daniel's preparation for the greater things God had in store for him. Daniel did not realize this at that time. He was, however, rewarded many times for his sacrifice in denying himself the natural corruptible things. Yet these denials of self were a physical blessing to him. Many things that seem a hardship to us are actually what we need, and prove to be blessings in disguise.

Some folk will say Daniel paid too much attention to the natural things. I have had people say my articles on FASTING contained too much about the natural, but let us see. A person never comes to God except he first comes in the natural, and then in the spiritual. A sinner first makes a natural step toward God before he gets saved. First, he kneels in the natural after he is convicted, then he opens his lips naturally to start a prayer to God. The breath that he breathes to God is natural, his voice is natural, in that he cries out to God in confession as he surrenders his all to God for acceptance; he yields all of his natural powers to God before the spiritual new birth takes place. There are many natural steps taken by the sinner in order to experience the spiritual new birth, whereas free salvation is one supernatural act of God. No one can come to God, saved or unsaved, for any need, large or small, without coming first to God in the natural. The first words of a prayer are usually too natural to be heard by Jesus. However, in a short time, the worship is transformed, and if a person really has his heart in it he begins worshiping God in "spirit and in truth." When a fast is undertaken it starts in the natural and ends in the spiritual. Natural things in their proper places do play a great part when consecrated to God in drawing us into the spiritual. Jesus Christ knew this of course; in studying His sayings and teachings, we find He spoke more about wealth and that which pertains to food and eating than about anything else in His ministry. God's three foundations of giving, prayer, and fasting, will make balanced Christians.

A CALL TO FASTING FOR NATIONAL REPENTANCE

Daniel 9:3: "And I set my face unto the Lord God, to seek by PRAYER and SUPPLICATIONS, WITH FASTING, and SACK CLOTH, and ASHES:"

DANIEL observed all of these NATURAL THINGS and entered into the deeper prayer of FASTING to prevail upon God for Israel, even placing himself as an unrighteous person along with his people. "We have sinned, and have committed iniquity, and have done wickedly, and have rebelled, even by departing from thy precepts and from thy judgments." Daniel 9:5. Daniel's prayer and confession is one of the greatest prayers recorded. Daniel 9:3-20.

It concerned one of the greatest prophecies recorded in the Word. Daniel 9:20-27.

Yes, prophecies and great revelations are the results of FASTING AND PRAYER. Today God is no respecter of persons. A person can fast and set his heart toward God and receive understanding of prophecy and have great understanding of the Word. To have a prophet's experience, go into a prophet's-length fast.

In this manner was Daniel's FAST answered: "And while I was speaking, and praying, and confessing my sin and the sin of my people Israel, and presenting my supplication before the Lord my God for the holy mountain of my God: Yea, whiles I was speaking in prayer, even the man Gabriel whom I had seen in the vision at the beginning, being caused to fly swiftly, touched me about the time of the evening oblation. And he informed me, and talked with me, and said, O Daniel, I am now come forth to give thee skill and understanding. At the beginning of thy supplications the commandment came forth, and I am come to show thee; *for thou art greatly beloved*: therefore understand the matter, and consider the vision." Daniel 9:20-23.

I am not taking up the study of the vision here, but wish to state that it concerned many years of history of the children of Israel, and the remaining years of this dispensation, the time of Christ's second coming, and the great tribulation that will be poured upon the world.

Men and women are lost and are going to hell. Too few of us have the burden for souls that we ought to have.

Daniel was in repentance and heavy travail for a national repentance. He felt the pull and the burden, consequently he went the limit. He used the most effective method known in his time, and the most effective means known today, to intercede for his people who were lost. This was FASTING AND PRAYER. He had been studying the books of the prophets, the writings of Moses, and the other scriptures. He found that if his people would repent, restoration would begin. Daniel 9:2-19. Daniel even placed himself before God as a sinner. "We have sinned." Daniel 9:5.

As Christian men and women who love our Lord Jesus Christ, if we do not have a burden for souls as we should have, by all means let us ask God to give us such a burden.

FASTING MOTHER OF A FASTING FAMILY

"When I was twenty-two, the Lord gave me a Christian husband. I helped my husband in mission, hospital, and prison work. The Lord gave us a lovely daughter, Mary Ann, and later I asked God for a son. My husband fasted fourteen days and the soul of Little David was given to us. He was born nine months after the fourteen day fast.

"When David was five years old I fasted seven days for God to heal him of an eye disease. This disease was so serious, Little David had to be led as one blind. At the completion of my fast of seven days and Little David's fast of three days, God not only healed but baptized him with the Holy Ghost.

"I little knew at that time, that four years later, Little David would begin the ministry through which thousands of souls accepted Christ. I sit in rap t attention as the Holy Spirit takes over the fleshly body that God favored me to bring forth in this world, being fully assured that a little boy could not perform the miracles as Little David does unless directed by the Holy Spirit.

"I am sure if every mother would fast and pray before and after the birth of her children, there would be no juvenile delinquency and no divorces, but rather obedient children and unbroken homes.

"My husband recently fasted eighteen days, Mary Ann fasted twelve days, and I fasted ten days for our future revival campaign. The results immediately following were miraculous. My husband had many prayers answered and some of the greatest meetings we have ever had came after these fasts. As high as twelve thousand people came out in one service and hundreds were converted.

Sister Gertrude Walker"

NEVER HEARD A SERMON IN ENGLAND
ON FASTING

"Dear Brother in Christ:

I received some of your tracts on fasting and prayer and a report of your book, entitled 'Atomic Power With God.' After reading the tracts I learned how to fast and can say that it does GIVE ONE ATOMIC POWER WITH GOD.

I have been interested in fasting for some time now, but until I received your tracts thru the HERALD OF HIS COMING, I knew very little about it. I regret to say that I have never heard a sermon in my life on fasting. I am desperate about the condition of the CHURCH OF CHRIST. It is so powerless. I too intend to fast more so I can have more power with God.

I have enclosed a ten shilling note to cover cost of 'Atomic Power With God.' If there is any left over, please make it up by enclosing some tracts.

Yours truly,
A sinner saved by grace,
Pastor F. H."
Wednesbury,
South Staffs, England

Chapter VI

THE PLAIN SIMPLE TEACHINGS OF CHRIST

"Labour not for the meat which perisheth, but *for that meat which endureth unto everlasting life,* which the Son of man shall give unto you:" John 6:27.

"FEED ME WITH FOOD CONVENIENT FOR ME: LEST I BE FULL, AND DENY THEE." Proverbs 30: 8, 9.

The human body God gave to man may be properly fed with "FOOD CONVENIENT FOR IT" and with the elements that are required for perfect nourishment. But the prevailing methods of feeding the body, with materials that are foreign to it, must of necessity weaken, irritate and sicken it.

Although God has provided the source of supply for all the faculties of the body, there is every reason for feeding our bodies with the same intelligence as is shown by experts who raise flowers or live stock. There should be as much common sense shown in one case as in the others.

Today, human thinking is on so low a plane that man gives careful attention to the health of livestock and pets, and seeks to prevent rather than cure diseases among them, yet IGNORES THE SAME NEED FOR HUMAN BEINGS. Florists feed plants with the exact foods they need, and with air and sunshine as required, whereas human beings are not given two percent of that care. Much of the food that is fed to the human body is a burden to it rather than a "CONVENIENCE," Furthermore humanity lacks the mental initiative to take steps to correct this evil. The average Christian abuses, neglects and ignores the vital welfare of the temple of the Holy Ghost.

The more one "LABOURS" about "THE MEAT" and seasons his food with fancy flavorings, sauces, and condiments, the more harmful it becomes to his already over stimulated organs. This certainly cannot be pleasing

to our Master's will. All through the Word of God we are
taught the plain, unadulterated truth of simplicity. An
over-extended menu cannot be an asset to the child of God
to PRODUCE FAITH and good works for the Master.

The human body consists of a food-cavity, a head, two
arms and two legs, all housed in skin framed upon bones.
The food-cavity begins at the mouth, bulges at the
stomach, and continues for many yards to its end. All
the organs of the body are satellites of the food-cavity.
The mouth is the upper end of the food-cavity: and it so
far masters the mind that the latter becomes its slave.
This food-cavity, with its many demands for attention,
practically rules the life of nearly every human being.

DOES THE FOOD HABIT HAVE YOU? DO YOU
HAVE CONTROL OF THE FOOD?

When a person goes on even a few days fast, he can
definitely decide to which of these questions he answers,
"yes." Sad to say, in most cases the individual seldom
gets far on the fast before he faints, and has to agree re-
luctantly that he is a SLAVE OF FOOD.

In these United States, more than a billion dollars
a month are spent for an excess of food which is useless,
wasteful, and injurious, and is the enemy of mind and body.
Man will not follow the plain common sense teachings of
Jesus Christ upon this subject and act upon them. The
high cost of living goes right on up, and it is nothing more
than the cost of WRONG LIVING. The trusts that force
prices up are merely taking advantage of the dis-TRUST
in GOD.

There are four main basic health foods given to man. If
these four plain, natural, health-building foods were relied
upon more and used simply, in their natural form, there
would be better health and greater freedom from disease
for almost everyone. These four complete foods are practically as life-giving as the blood itself. They are:

1. FRUIT
2. MILK
3. VEGETABLES — CEREALS
4. EGGS

The whole nation knows too little of what it should
know about food. God's people know even less, and in
consequence they are continually coming to God for heal-

SIMPLE TEACHINGS OF CHRIST   125

ing while all they need is a little knowledge about food
and eating. "MY PEOPLE ARE DESTROYED FOR
LACK OF KNOWLEDGE." Hosea 4:6.

But, strange to say, man is still groping in the darkness of almost total ignorance of what are foods and what
are not foods for his body. In every generation since the
birth of life on earth, nearly one hundred percent of
humanity has paid the heavy penalty for lack of knowledge by unnecessary suffering and untimely death; and it
should be the goal of every Christian, to see to it that the
temple of the Holy Spirit is cared for as well and properly
as we care for any other department of our life.

"As soon as Zion *travailed, she brought forth her
children*". Isaiah 66:8. There is nothing America needs
more than a national revival. When will we have one?
When Christian people get down to business with God
and TRAVAIL. The greatest travail possible after a
person has God's Spirit in his heart, is through Fasting
and Prayer. FASTING is travail that will reach higher
than any other. It is the greatest travail that can be
brought about. It is the TRAVAIL PRAYER. Daniel
realized the value of the travailing prayer and utilized it
to the fullest extent.

Thank God that many Christians are now fasting ten
days, twenty-one days, and even forty days. More Christians are fasting now in America, and throughout the
world than at any other time since the time of Christ.
The author has been speaking to many thousands of
people in the largest auditoriums available, and has crack-
ed down upon the flesh and given the full truth of fasting
to many of God's people who heretofore never knew what
a fast of more than several days was like. This last day
message is Bible prophecy being fulfilled before our eyes.
(See Joel 1:14. 15; 2: 12-18).

In Portland, Oregon, the author spoke in the Civic
Auditorium which seats five thousand people. Nearly
every seat was filled. A continuous fasting chain was started
in one of the churches and it is going on at this time.

Little David, twelve year old boy evangelist, preached
the evangelistic sermon and scores of persons were converted and scores of others were filled with the Spirit and
healed. (See photo elsewhere in book).

The Salem, Oregon, Senior High School auditorium was

filled, and hundreds had to be turned away. The author spoke, and taught on the prophet's-length fast and hundreds of ministers and thousands of people were thrilled to learn of the protracted consecration fast. Scores of folk started fasting for an old-time major national revival. (See picture of the high school auditorium.) In the State of Washington, the author secured six such high schools where the entire Gospel was preached under the power and anointing of the Holy Spirit.

Our large fasting evangelistic party and myself, usually go into the city campaigns on neutral grounds, and on an inter-denominational basis, but in Salem, Rev. Walter S. Frederick, pastor of the large Assembly of God church wanted to sponsor the campaign in his city. Rev. E. S. Williams, Chairman of the General Council of the Assemblies of God, Springfield, Missouri, opened a Bible Conference in conjunction with the District Council at the conclusion of our campaign.

We finally consented to go to Salem. Reverend Frederick's church was too small to accommodate the crowd, although it seated over six hundred.

Surely the Lord cannot turn a deaf ear to the deep praying and travail of his people and there must be a revival of power, of salvation, of healings, and of miracles.

In the tenth chapter of Daniel, he again went before the Lord for "three full weeks." "Daniel alone saw the vision." His comrades did not see the great vision, which concerned the very days in which we are now living, because Daniel alone had fasted these days. Daniel was determined to get his prayers through. He never fainted or gave up when he sought the Lord. This shows great faith. Not only was Daniel blessed in getting the answer to his petitions, but he also received added rewards for his fastings. He was privileged to see ahead of time the Son of man in His glorified body.

"From the first day that thou didst set thine heart to understand, and to *chasten* thyself before thy God, thy words were heard." Dan. 10:12.

Then an explanation was given as to why the answer to his fast and prayer was not received from the first. This is why one should not be discouraged or become faithless when his prayers are not answered from the first.

Daniel wanted a revelation and more light on prop-

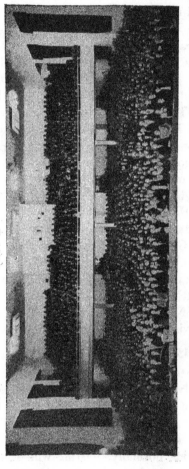

Senior High School Auditorium, Salem, Oregon, Jan. 19, 1947—126 sinners came forward to Jesus this day. Results of the "prophets-length FASTS." After 2000 people packed the building, the fire department was called to lock the doors to prevent others from storming in. The large Assembly of God church proved too small, so Pastor W. S. Frederick secured the largest auditorium in the city. This preceded the Northwest General Council Convention. Dr. E. S. Williams, of Springfield, and chairman, led the convention in a Bible conference in the First Methodist Church after Little David, boy preacher, and author were through this campaign. All denominations cooperated and hundreds of ministers were hungry f or old time fasting and prayer. The Presbyters voted acceptance of "Atomic Power With God Thru Fasting and Prayer." Many ministers were happy to learn about the prophet's-length fast.

hecy. Gabriel was the prophetic angel and he came to deliver the interpretation, "skill and understanding," but there were hindrances. Gabriel was no warrior angel, and could not overcome the Satanic powers. Michael was the fighting angel and had to come to the rescue. Where Michael is found, trouble is found. Michael did come, and he overcame all forces of evil so the great prophetic message of Gabriel concerning the end time, could get through.

This is a great chapter in the book of Daniel and should encourage us to have more faith, and to hold on to the promise of God as Daniel did. Daniel's great faith was largely a product of his FASTINGS.

Please note that FASTING IS A METHOD OF SELF- CHASTISEMENT. When we go down in fasting, other sad and bereaving experiences that may be to us a chastening from God's Hand, are frequently prevented just because we go after the Lord and touch Him in so precious a manner. Without frequent fastings, the continued eating habit becomes a destroyer of faith and the works of the Holy Spirit.

Our greatest goal in life should be, to be men and women after God's own heart. We should have a great burden for souls, seeking to turn many to righteousness. "They that be wise shall SHINE AS THE BRIGHTNESS OF THE FIRMAMENT: and they that turn many to RIGHTEOUSNESS as the stars for ever and ever." Daniel 12:3. "Be ye wise as serpents and harmless as doves".

FASTING SENSE

Waste material accumulates under the skin and turns to pus. It's only means of exit is to break through the skin in the form of pimples. To overcome this condition we must give the skin a chance to breathe. We must have the intestinal tract clean. We must have kidneys and lungs functioning normally. Fasting will bring this about. Girls have taken a fast of a few days and have come out without pimples, and have received a beautiful complexion. God's young people can have the finest natural complexions as a result of fasting.

When eating, the lungs, the skin, the kidneys, and the colon eliminate approximately two pounds of waste each, a day. When fasting, each organ eliminates approximately the same proportion of a reduced quantity. The pollution, however, is far more poisonous and more burdensome.

Meat gives quick energy, but only because it requires a fast working body to take care of it. It is only through the stimulation and over-activity of the body while trying to take care of the meat that one seems to feel better. Every organ is working fast, consequently more blood is supplied to the different organs of the body. This gives us pep, so to speak, but in the long run it is depleting our energy. It is a form of false stimulation.

Upton Sinclair, speaking on the subject of fasting states: "I have discovered for myself the value of fasting. I have learned what nonsense it is to talk about the danger of starving to death as a result of fasting."

I am giving a couple of cases of extremes in fasting. Mr. Jedisiel Laib of Grodno, Poland, fasted six days a week for thirty years. Each Saturday he had whole grain bread and water.

Dr. Bernard Jensen of Santa Barbara, Calif., tells in his book:

"A young woman seventeen years old, by the name of Maria De Conceises, from Mendes, Brazil, fasted 180 days, or six months. She recovered from the epilepsy with which she was afflicted. There was no great loss of weight, she remained very active, and physicians found all organs perfect after the fast." If true, it is the longest fast ever recorded.

Fasting is a method of preparing the body to take food.

Most ordinary and some major ailments will respond naturally to fasting. Purifying the blood stream will enable it to take up waste material floating around in the body, give it a good house-cleaning, carry material deposited in various parts of the body to the eliminative organs which will then be able to handle it.

No matter how young or old a Christian may be, fasting will help him physically and spiritually.

I am not a vegetarian, but I am interested in abstemious living for the glory of God. Research shows the meat-eating Indians lived about sixty years while the nut and maize-eating Indians reached the mature age of one hundred-six to one hundred eighty (Estes).

More than two million persons are sick abed every day in the year in these United States of America. Christians, let us have a burden for the sick and afflicted as well as for sinners. Divine healing will often bring a sinner to Christ.

Over 800,000 people will die this year from preventable diseases.

The tobacco expense, direct and indirect, is greater than the cost of the United States Government.

In ancient times the soldiers of Sparta ate but one meal a day.

Feeding a sick person to keep up his strength is the surest way to kill him.

A person can live longer by fasting than on white bread and water.

It is said that more blood is shed on the operating table than on the battlefield.

It is possible to starve to death with a full stomach.

The primary need of the body is oxygen, not food. Dr. Arthur Vos makes the statement that ninety percent of all food required by the body must be oxygen. More than fifty percent of the weight of a human being is oxygen. If the oxygen contained in his body were set free, it is estimated it would fill 750 cubic feet of space.

Suicides have increased 600 percent in the last seventy years.

Two hundred fifty thousand American women yearly enter the shadows of motherhood unfit to bring children into the world.

One person out of every six, suffers a spell of sickness during each year.

27,400 people at home today will be obliged to enter a hospital tomorrow.

For the glory and honor of Jesus Christ, fast and get into the SPIRITUAL. It exalts, praises, and pleases the ONE who bought us with a price. Any way, we are not our own, so why fail to endure a few days discomfort in fasting, when we can be so very much helped in so many ways?

A Thousand Converted

The Little David Evangelistic party consisted of Little David, 12 year old boy preacher, his sister Mary Ann who recently concluded a ten day fast, Little David's father, Rev. Jack Walker, who also fasted ten days, Little

David's mother and little sister Esther Sharon, age 2, and the Rose of Sharon Trio, the Gering sisters, Gladys, Joyce, and Jo Anne, who are consecrated girl singers from Spokane, Washington. Jo Anne recently fasted ten days. Miss Gladys Gering fasted fourteen days. Miss Joyce Gering fasted twenty-one days. Other members of this large party were Evangelists Dale and Barbara Hanson, —they fasted twenty-eight days and received a powerful anointing for additional service to Jesus Christ. This large group, with the author and family, made up the RE-VIVAL PARTY.

We went to Denver for one week. We had one night stands in various churches.

We went into Brother Sanders' Calvary Church for the afternoon special teaching on Fasting. Many ministers, including Reverend Muncy, Overseer of the Church of God, attended the classes. Over two hundred people joined in the fast, and several continuous fasting chains were organized.

All the pastors welcomed fasting and prayer for an old-time revival.

The evening services were packed out in every church. MORE THAN FOUR HUNDRED SOUGHT GOD AT AN OLD FASHIONED ALTAR IN THE CITY OF DENVER. Many said it was the city's greatest revival.

We left Denver for Council Bluffs, Iowa, where Brother Ted Fitch rented the city auditorium. The Foursquare Church in Omaha under Chaplain Musgroves made it possible to have a great revival meeting in both Council Bluffs and Omaha. Chaplain Musgroves' Foursquare Church was packed out. The Lord wonderfully blessed and approximately three hundred were converted in this area in about five days. A continuous fasting chain was started with fifty people fasting when we left—some went twenty-one days.

We came Des Moines from Omaha to the large Foursquare Tabernacle where Rev. Caswell is Pastor. Large crowds attended the afternoon services on the teaching of the FASTING PRAYER. The evening services were also packed out and some were turned away.

We went into the Hoyt Sherman Auditorium seating 1600. Several additional hundreds were standing and at least 500 were turned away. Three hundred were converted and really cried out to God in tears for salvation in the six days we were there. A hundred went to fasting and praying for longer than they had ever fasted in their lives.

A fasting chain was started with 50 persons fasting as we left Des Moines for Chicago where the auditorium was also packed out and hundreds converted.

At least a thousand souls were converted in these three very short meetings, in Denver, Omaha and Des Moines.

WHY FASTING IS UNPOPULAR

Fasting is the threshold of FAITH. It does not seem as if it could profit one. People go too much by feeling. When in the fast proper this very feeling of emptiness and self-insufficiency is FAITH IN ITSELF because doubt is being destroyed. Most of the weaknesses of the fast are actually making faith. Faith is built up on the things that seem as nothing and of that which cannot be seen, therefore the FAST is actually faith itself when it is dedicated and consecrated to the Lord Jesus.

Many persons, including many ministers, started fasting in the city of Denver, Colo.

Here are several testimonies:

"I am so happy that I can now seek the Lord in a greater manner then I previously have known.

"I am ten days along in a fast. Before fasting I had asthma so badly that I was miserable most of the time. Jesus came and healed me completely on the sixth day of fasting. I am so happy, and I rejoice that He has been so very real and precious to me in this fast. I have attained heights of joy and gladness I never before realized was possible.

"My fast is turning out exactly like the book, 'Atomic Power with God' teaches. About the third day my hunger left. Now I am over my weakness, and I feel stronger than I have ever felt in my life.

"I have lost thirteen pounds and hope to fast at least fourteen days. I have four more days to go and I feel better spiritually than I have ever felt in my life."

Sister L. J.
Denver, Colo.

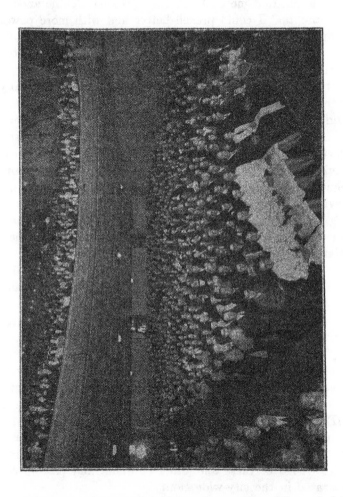

Hoyt-Sherman Auditorium, Des Moines, Ia. — Many folks pushed their way into the auditorium after every seat had been filled. Six hundred people had to be turned away in this FASTING PRAYER REVIVAL.

We first went into the large Foursquare tabernacle of Brother Caswell. It was crowded out every evening. Great crowds also attended the specialized teaching on the FASTING PRAYER in the afternoons, including many ministers. Many different denominations cooperated in this city wide meeting. More than three hundred came forward to accept Christ and hundreds of folks received the light on the major Bible protracted FASTING. Part of crowd shown.

"I am pastor of Calvary Church (Assembly of God) in the city of Denver. I bought Dr. Fanklin Hall's book on the consecration fast and after fasting only seven days, I felt better than I had felt for years. The members of my church told me that this fast gave me double anointing and that I could preach better and with more power than I had ever preached previously.

"When Dr. Hall came to the city of Denver, I invited him to my church for special teaching on the subject of fasting. Scores of folks started fasting and I can say many were healed and saved. I fasted two weeks at this time, and secured greater results with the Lord than ever before.

"Brother Hall came in advance of the evangelistic party, and got a lot of persons to pray and fast for a great revival. After the large party came to Denver many churches closed including my own, and one of the greatest revivals the city of Denver has ever seen came through fasting and prayer. Approximately four hundred people came forward to accept Jesus Christ in old-time repentance. Many were healed and blessed in other ways.

"We now have a continuous fasting chain in our church. Several other churches also have a fasting chain, to go on continually until Jesus comes.

"Many ministers also became interested in the protracted consecration fast, including Reverend Hamilton of the FOUR SQUARE CHURCH, Reverend Belk of the Radio Prayer League Church, Reverend Muncy, overseer of the Church of God, Reverend Rolls of the Englewood Assembly of God church, Reverend Cooper of the DENVER REVIVAL TABERNACLE, Reverend McClure of the beautiful Central Assembly, Calvary Church of which I am pastor, and several other churches and pastors. All of these and other churches and pastors cooperated in the city-wide campaign.

"Hereafter, every Tuesday evening we are giving a special Bible study on the consecration fast. Our church accepts fasting, and we are hungry to go into deeper fastings and prayer to see the spiritual gifts restored."

Brother Sanders,

Denver, Colorado

Please see auditorium picture of The Denver Revival

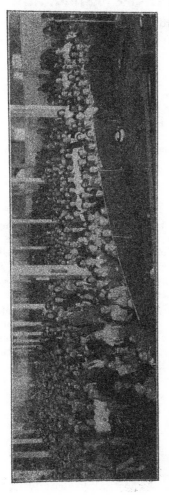

Fasting and prayer revival, Denver, Colo. Ten Churches came together to have a city wide campaign. Some of the Churches were, The Radio Prayer League, Calvary Tabernacle, Englewood Assembly, Central Assembly, Foursquare, Church of God, Missionary Alliance, and The Denver Revival Tabernacle where the above photograph was taken in one of the afternoon services. Hundreds were turned away. Over 400 came forward in the eight days we were in Denver. Two weeks before campaign, a continuous fasting chain was started.

Tabernacle where hundreds were turned away. This was typical of the crowds at all revival services held in Denver. The success of this revival was definitely attributed to THE TRAVAIL PRAYER OF FASTING FOR SOULS TO BE CONVERTED.

A BELLY SERVER BEFORE FASTING, NOW FREE

Many of the Lord's people are healed and have an experience such as is given in the first part of the testimony of a lady who fasted twenty-one days.

"I have had many healings from the Lord in the last twenty-three years. I now have a long standing case of hyper acidity that I have not been able to heal. Brother Kelso prayed for me at the tent meeting that he was holding in East Los Angeles. The Lord touched my body and I received a partial healing, only to FIND OUT AFTERWARD I HAD AN ABNORMAL APPETITE. THIS WAS THE MOST FEROCIOUS APPETITE THAT I EVER HAD. I COULD EAT ANY AND EVERYTHING. IT SEEMED THAT I COULD NOT CONTROL IT AT ALL. IT CONTROLLED ME.

I prayed much for help and in answer to prayer, a book called "Atomic Power With God", was placed in my hands. After reading only two chapters, I started fasting because I realized that my trouble WAS THE LOVE OF FOOD. I asked the Lord to forgive me my sins of intemperance. After fifteen days of fasting I began feeling better, my sinusitis left my body and a few days later I felt better than I have felt in many years.

I first heard about your book at Evangelist Dale and Barbara Hanson's large tent revival where many were converted. They were getting many folk to start fasting ten and twenty-one days. I have won many victories thru prayer and fasting, now I can go into the longer Bible fasts. With the information contained in the book it seems so much easier to fast.

Sister A. N."

Montebello, Calif.

I consider this an important letter of testimony and confession. In it one can readily understand why many of the Lord's children are not healed. I cannot feel that the Lord will heal His people only to yield to the flesh and the devil. Fastings will help undo sins of intemperance.

Chapter VII

FASTING BECOMES FAITH
RECEIVING SPIRITUAL GIFTS

"FAITH IS THE SUBSTANCE OF THINGS HOPED FOR, THE EVIDENCE OF THINGS NOT SEEN. For by it the elders obtained a good report. Through faith we UNDERSTAND THAT THE WORLDS WERE FRAMED BY THE WORD OF GOD, SO THAT THINGS WHICH ARE SEEN WERE NOT MADE OF THINGS WHICH DO APPEAR." Heb. 11:1-3.

If we are to receive healings and answers to our prayers it is most essential that we have faith, not only faith to be healed, but FAITH IN GOD and in all that He stands for. We must have FAITH in an INVISIBLE GOD, a God that cannot be seen. "Who dwelleth in the light, unapproachable, whom no man hath seen or can see." 1 Tim. 6:16. John said, "No man hath seen God at any time." John 1:18.

God is an infinite Being, existing on a plane so high and far above us that "as the heavens are far above the earth, so are His thoughts above our thoughts and His ways above our ways." Is. 55:8. We have to have FAITH "to please Him." Heb. 11:6. "He that cometh to God must BELIEVE THAT HE IS, and that HE IS A REWARDER OF THEM THAT DILIGENTLY SEEK HIM. Without a *SPECIAL PRAYER OR FASTING EXPERIENCE* our thoughts, our finite minds are absolutely incapable of grasping HIM. Likewise our sense of seeing, hearing, smelling, tasting, and feeling cannot in any way receive any impression of Him. We cannot detect His presence except as He desires it, and He would reveal Himself through a FASTING AND PRAYER EXPERIENCE. God is a hidden Personality so far as we are concerned, and One who will always remain hidden except as He desires to come out of His hiding place. Fasting and prayer will draw HIM out. We cannot reach out and touch Him, but HE WILL REACH DOWN AND

TOUCH US MORE READILY IN RESPONSE TO THE
FASTING PRAYER.

To accomplish our fullest objective in the consecration fast, there are three special zones that *must* be contacted. The focus of our entire consciousness should be
directed thereon to bring the necessary factors together
to insure success in the attainment of a "gift" of the
Spirit or other vital needs sought. They are: (1) a deep
burden for the object sought; (2) ourself in deep consecration, yieldedness and humility, and last but most important (3) the fullest realization that Jesus is God, and
He is capable and willing to grant the petition as soon as
He sees your faith in Him and His power. Since this is the
most important zone to be contacted, we are giving it
special attention for your fullest illumination.

The human mind, due to so much carnality, fleshly
lusts, and abnormal appetites, finds it very difficult to form
any impression or idea of an infinite invisible being. Man
wants to see and feel what he deals with. He wants something tangible. Israel found it very difficult to worship
their great GOD—because they could not see Him. They
refused to go on a fast in order to come close to HIM.
(Deut. 8:3). But they found no trouble at all to worship
the gods of the Canaanites, whose images they could see
and feel. The heathen of today worship spirits, but they
must make images of these spirits.

THE SUBSTANCE OF GOD

To surmount this difficulty, God made an image of
Himself, a tangible image that man could put his hands
on—could see with his eyes and hear with his ears. God
originally made man after His own image (Gen. 1:26), so
man must be the image of God. This image He made
(Christ) must look like man and have human form and
characteristics. Heb. 1:3: "The express image of His
person" or "the very image of His substance." God did
not look the universe over and choose something that He
created, but He took of Himself. He used His own substance. If He had used anything else, then the Son would
be a created being. But as God is eternal and His substance is eternal, therefore the Son has existed from eterni-
ty. He is not the first created, but He is "the first-born of
all creation." Col. 1:15.

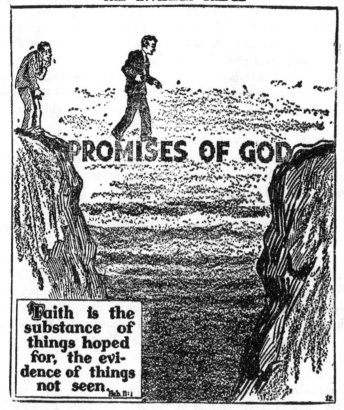

PROMISES OF GOD

Faith is the substance of things hoped for, the evidence of things not seen. Heb 11:1

Although prayer alone will develop some FAITH, the full and complete formula of Jesus must be followed out completely to have the faith that removes mountains. The great faith producer is found in Matthew 17:21. The consecrated FAST is a step into faith. A faith that takes hold and makes spiritual giants out of weak humans. It takes the props out from under us. The main prop upon which we lean so strongly is food. Finally the participant finds that he is leaning only on Jesus in the middle of faith, and fasting has become faith. A gift becomes within our reach.

The FASTING experience will give us the FAITH to DISCOVER MORE INTIMATELY and COMPLETELY WHAT THE SON IS LIKE. 1 John 1:5 says, "GOD is LIGHT," therefore, the substance of God is light-giving. When God talked to Moses from the bush, Moses saw fire. Later on Moses came face to face with God by food abstention for forty days. No wonder for "He dwelleth in the light unapproachable." Consequently, the SON also radiates LIGHT. When He was transfigured on the mount they saw a SHINING LIGHT. Luke 9:28-36.

This light that shines forth from the Son is not a reflected nor a borrowed light as the moon reflects the sun's light. The SON being made of the Father's light-giving substance, He radiates His own light.

The substance of God is also life-giving. This is more clearly realized after several weeks of fasting. (John 5:26) God can impart life. Existence is one thing while *life is something different*. This life-giving substance when placed in the Son also makes Him a life-giver. (John 5:21; 5:26.) When the Son spoke to the widow's dead son, he sat up and spoke. When He spoke to the dead young woman she arose. When He cried, "Lazarus, come forth," the dead, decaying, vile-smelling body became a living man, because in the Son was life and He could give it unto whom He pleased. However, even before the Life-giver had these manifestations, and before He imparted life, it was necessary that even He should have the FASTING PRAYER experience of forty days, plus HIS TEMPTATION.

"God gave unto us eternal life and this life is in His son. 1 John 5:11. Just what benefit is that to us? "Whoso hath the Son hath the LIFE." HALLELUJAH! Men are dead in trespasses and sins and God wants to make them alive. So He takes His own life-giving substance and puts it into His SON. Then He says, "Kindly accept my SON if you want eternal LIFE." This makes the SON the necssary link between humanity and God. It is the "only Name under heaven" by which man can be saved. Acts 4:12. The devil stole eternal life from man in the begining by tempting him through his appetites and getting him to EAT WRONG FOOD. Jesus has come to bring LIFE BACK: not by eating "bread alone" but by "the words of God". We live by partaking of THE SUBSTANCE OF GOD. The SUBSTANCE OF GOD IMPARTS LIFE

WHEREVER IT GOES. When we eat and absorb the Son of God's substance, we receive eternal life because the LIFE-GIVER ENTERS. ETERNAL LIFE does not begin after we die. We have it now while we are in this flesh and bone tabernacle, because we possess "Christ in you" Gal. 4:19. Eternal life remains as long as "Christ in you" remains.

The name of God, "Jehovah" or "Jaweh," imparts the idea of His being self-supporting and self-sufficient. Therefore, the substance of God must be eternal and immutable. This means that God always has been and always will be, and time does not change Him. We humans are dependent upon the four great essentials—air, water, sleep, and food, to maintain our life processes. Remove these and life soon ceases. We are subject to the ravages of time, and age leaves it's mark. With God it is different. His substance needs no imparting of energy from an outside source. He does not need air, food or sunshine. He keeps right on existing, without help. Time, ages upon ages, does not change HIM. If He needed help where would He apply for it? Who would give it to Him? Jesus said, "I AM THE BREAD OF LIFE." God's food or substance gives energy continuously, without diminishing in volume or becoming weaker. This must be a wonderful food. Let us try living on it more often. There is none like it in the whole universe. He is the only God and beside Him there is none other. No wonder He becomes jealous when demons and men claim to be deity and take unto themselves worship that belongs to Him. Likewise, is it any wonder that we cannot fully partake of His presence and the illumination of FAITH that is so necessary, except as we surrender for a time the things of the world. Abstain from FOOD and go into a FAST, then all other carnal and greedy appetites are vanquished by the speediest and most sucessful method known. This richer food, the word of God, (or substance of God) becomes a greater reality and the very God of heaven comes within our reach. It is not at all surprising that the glory of His Image is so tremendous that many stand in awe before Him. Man becomes so insignificant and Christ so highly magnified and glorified, that this new experience will be just the beginning of scores of like experiences in FASTING that will impart super FAITH IN CHRIST. Answered prayer then can be an accomplished fact, and that which heretofore seemed dead, will be an experience of SUPER ATOMIC LIFE AND POWER WITH GOD.

It is our purpose to EXALT JESUS CHRIST and to emphasize the importance of getting a real glimpse of HIM. We cannot have true faith unless we do see HIM and taste of the BREAD OF LIFE. Every conversion, every healing, and every prayer that has ever been answered has only come about by contacting Him and this had to be by FAITH. We are stressing the fact that a *major fasting experience* will more quickly produce that FAITH and that we may have such CONTACT WITH HIM that our sicknesses, afflictions and sorrows may be removed. "The effectual FERVENT PRAYER of a righteous man availeth much." James 5:16. There is no prayer so "effectual", so "fervent," as the FASTING PRAYER. To the consecrated Christian, the "FAST" is prayer.

The fasting prayer is the best way to get CLOSER to JESUS. It opens the way to receive spiritual gifts.

A sister from North Hollywood writes regarding her sixteen-day fast.

"Dear Brothers and Sisters in Christ:

I have been saved and have received the Holy Spirit. I wish to say that there is much more in store for you if you just try out this fasting prayer experience. It would make the Holy Spirit more real. On the third day of my sixteen-day fast, I received a call to be a missionary to Mexico. Jesus became more real to me than ever before. I am by nature a shy person and it was very hard for me to testify, but during the fast, the Lord took all of this stage fright away. FASTING and PRAYING IS THE BEST WAY THAT I KNOW OF TO BE DRAWN CLOSER TO THE LORD. Already I am seeing my prayers answered. The longer you fast the easier it is.

Your sister in Christ,

Miss Ellen Davis,
No. Hollywood, Calif.

When we get close to God we have VICTORY. Victory is a wonderful word. I love the sound of it. It means overcoming opposing forces. It means conquering enemies.

May God inspire us anew in BELIEVING that His victory, His triumph in this old world is certain! From the beginning of the Book to the end is a record of conflict—Satan and his agents in opposition to God and His people, but the children of God today, as the men of old, can be brought forth victoriously with a PRAYER-FASTING EXPERIENCE. This gives us the FAITH that will bring absolute deliverance through unconditional surrender to Jesus Christ in every way. "This is the VICTORY that overcomes the world, EVEN OUR FAITH." Even our faith! There must be definite, active faith in the triumph of our Christ, a faith that lays hold upon and claims His VICTORY over Satan. There must be determined, persistent faith that appropriates the promises and continually counts on what Jesus Christ the Lord offers us. It is a faith which actually rests upon the conviction that victory is ours through Jesus Christ. John 16:33; 1 Cor. 15:57.

Overcoming faith must express itself in PRAYER, for without prayer, faith becomes merely mental. The FASTING-PRAYER takes us out of this mental state by changing our environment completely from the natural to the spiritual. Prayer and FASTING as well as communion with God are vital to the child of God, for by this means he keeps that life connection so necessary to the victorious overcoming of all obstacles. As we go into this process, we become yielded vessels, and the good of our fellow-man is sought. This moves one out of self to see the need of others. It is faith that worketh by love. Gal. 5:6. There is no such thing as self-centeredness in a life of real overcoming. That is why many never know real victory in life. There is no real concern for others. Overcoming faith loves and seeks the glory of God. THE FASTING PRAYER GETS THE JOB DONE.

Overcoming faith takes heed of the light shining in a dark place. 2 Peter 1:19. A man with this overcoming faith sees the world getting darker, but he is not overcome, he is not thrown into dismay and despair; he knows the word of prophecy is being fulfilled. He knows that all the Lord has spoken will come to pass. He knows that day will dawn, and he is getting ready for flight. He who lives in this victory receives the warnings of God's Word to be ready for the coming of the Lord, and he is already separated in spirit from this world. Some day, perhaps soon,

He will share Christ's openly manifested victory over this world, the works of Satan, physical afflictions, weaknesses and sorrow.

One reason that fasting is not understood is because folk cannot feel and see what fasting is doing while fasting is in progress. Fasting is too much like FAITH. It leads one right up to the very threshold of faith itself. It is so nearly faith, that in one of the tracts I have written, I have called it "FAITH'S BROTHER." The consecration fast is so much like faith that it could almost be called FAITH. One reason fasting becomes faith is because it brings one face to face with the doubts and unbelief that must be removed before FAITH COMES IN. Before these can be removed, the individual must be brought up close enough to reach out and pull them out of the way. When our boys were in battle, they had to get close enough to the enemy to make a forceful enough contact to blast out the barriers that were in the way in order to have a clear pathway that would lead to certain victory. At times the cost was great, but victory was certain when the proper approach was made. Fasting will do this very thing in the spiritual warfare and will produce the FAITH if one does not faint and fall by the wayside. It produces because Jesus said it would. Matthew, chapter 17. People CAN-NOT UNDERSTAND FASTING UNLESS THEY FAST A WEEK OR MORE, AT LEAST.

A certain brother gave me this testimony:

"I have been working with the sick and afflicted; many times a demon-possessed individual would be left in my custody to patiently work and pray with. Many a one I was able to pray through and cast these demons out. When I secured the book 'Atomic Power With God,' I was determined that I would be used even more successfully by God in this calling. I began a consecration FAST UNTO GOD. After three days, hunger left me. I was able to carry on my regular work for two weeks. I then gave it up so that I could devote my time to more praying and meditation on the Lord. I gave myself to prayer but found it a great battle to pray like I should. I didn't feel that I was getting any place at times, however I knew that

God was working in a different manner than I ever had experienced before.

Many Scriptures and puzzling problems that had been obscure to me for a long time became very clear. A deeper understanding of God's word came to me like a great flash out of the clear blue skies. A new meaning to the Scriptures was realized. Prayers were answered. My hearing is better. I can see without glasses now.

After fasting twenty days I thought that hunger returned and broke the fast. Later I decided that it was only habit hunger, and after two days of fruit juices, I continued to fast. I really praise God for all the blesings that I received on the fast.

I have more faith, now, than ever."

Glen Gladon,
3920 N.E. 105th St.,
Portland, Ore.

Fasting gives surprising faith to a person although during the fast it seems that one is actually accomplishing less for God. When we battle the old man, many things do not seem oftentimes to be what they really are. That is, spiritually, one has made great progress, but in the natural it appears that he is defeated. He is *not* defeated, but actually, the "old man" that wars against the Spirit is conquered.

Everybody has a lap but our lap disappears when we stand up. Did you ever stop to think where your lap went to? At times the lap is very important. We never seem to bother about it, but if we did not have a lap we human beings would at times be in difficult straits. Your lap probably goes where the hole went in the doughnut that you took a bite out of, yet you never give a thought as to where the hole went.

Likewise doubts, fleshly lusts, and unbelief disappear in a major consecration fast. We should not let it bother us that we feel depressed, and miserable and weak in the flesh. We really should have such prayer-fasting experiences so frequently that we will learn to avoid analyzing every little feeling and trying to weigh things out. We should take Jesus at His word and concentrate on travail-

ing for souls. We may become so used to defeating the
devil by prayer and fasting, that the demons and hell will
tremble when we launch forth on this great crusade.
Spiritual success will follow as the night follows the day.
One reason folk do not fast is because fasting in itself is too
much like faith. It is the nearest thing to faith.

There are too many Christians standing still, and when
one stands still it is not long until he is going backward in
his Christian experience. When a person goes forward, he
never bothers to analyze every movement of his legs, he
just marches on to victory and to more victory. A person
actually becomes more tired standing than he does walking.
When walking each leg gets to rest one half of the time,
while standing still calls into operation nearly all of the
muscles of both legs and feet all of the time. Our Christian
experience is the same way: it is a lot easier to keep going,
to keep on the run by fasting and prayer than to try to
stand still. Keep going on and prevent backsliding. A
live Christian always keeps going on and on and never lets
up for one moment.

Evangelist Demetrios Kardassakis tells of the healing
of his wife in answer to prayer and fasting:

"My wife was five weeks in the Lane Hospital, San
Francisco, with cancer. As a last resort an operation was
advised. While she was on the operating table (four
hours), the doctors found the cancer (in the womb) in such
condition that they dared not operate on her. They were
afraid she would bleed to death or that blood poisoning
would set in and she would die in just a few hours. They
also told me that no man in the world could cure her.

"She was sent home and fasted twelve days without
any food. At five o'clock p.m., on the twelfth day of the
fast, some strangers came to my house and prayed for my
wife. In half an hour she asked for something to eat, and
was definitely and instantly healed, praise the Lord! When
the nurse came to check her, she could hardly believe that
she was the same woman. Later, her weight increased from
one hundred fifteen to one hundred thirty nine pounds. The
fourth month after the healing, the same doctors examined
her and found her in perfect health. Praise the Lord
forever."

I have a report in regard to a precious colored sister.
Sister Dabney makes prayer a business. She seldom sleeps

or eats. She seems to pray all day and all night. She has a real ministry of travail for souls. There is no foolishness about her, no, not even when visiting because she prays and travails for sinners constantly.

Sister Dabney made a vow to God that if He would send sinners to their church and save them, she would fast and pray three days and three nights each week, in the church, for two years, and continue to pray another year.

After she began this time of prayer and fasting, God began to work. Sinners were sent in and soon their hall, which had heretofore been empty, began filling up and was crowded out.

God finally led her to call regular 4.00 A.M. prayer meetings. About 350 people were there before the church each morning, a half hour ahead of time to enjoy the wonderful presence of the Lord. Everyone was overshadowed. Later on more than four hundred met at 4.00 o'clock in the morning to pray for the wicked city and for souls everywhere. The city was stirred! Think of how many souls are getting saved because men and women travail in these early hours of the morning before God. Sister Dabney's fasts and prayers have built up such faith that the fire of the Holy Spirit stirs both sinners and saints.

A report in the form of a letter tells of the very remarkable results in "The Garden of Prayer Church." Many have spent seventy-two hours in FASTING and PRAYER, and some have FASTED FOR TEN DAYS. In a five year period, eight thousand seventy-four souls have come to Jesus for salvation. Six thousand have been filled with the Spirit. Thousands have been healed and many others have received special answers to prayers. We are indeed thankful to the Lord for a fasting prayer warrior, like sister E. J. Dabney and her group of workers of Philadelphia.

When it comes to fasting, the colored race have put the lighter races to shame. Yes, the colored people have out-fasted the white folk. In the days of Azusa, forty years ago, the colored race was honored by an outpouring of the Holy Spirit. Why? The colored people fasted and prayed more than the white people so God let the latter rain outpouring of the Holy Spirit come through this humble race.

Remember, anyone can be a Daniel, an Elijah, or a

prophet, if they just meet certain conditions of God, regardless of race, or nationality. God is no respecter of persons. To have a prophet's experience, fast twenty-one to forty days. This should not seem strange to do.

GIFTS OF THE SPIRIT THROUGH FASTING

If it was necessary for Jesus to fast forty days in order to receive spiritual Gifts, how can we expect to receive them doing less, without following His pattern?

"THE MANIFESTATION OF THE SPIRIT IS GIVEN TO EVERY MAN TO PROFIT WITHAL." (I Cor. 12: 1-11).

In the study of consecrated fasting we have come to know that it is the greatest possible means of obtaining the favor of God and keeping filled with His Spirit.

The church of Jesus Christ has been circumvallated to fasting for so long that she is not accustomed to practicing and having in operation the gifts of the Spirit. When fasting is again accepted on a greater scale, which is surely a part of the "FAITH THAT WAS ONCE DELIVERED UNTO THE SAINTS," (Jude 3) it will not be long until the gifts will again appear in the church and in their proper place. The church has been praying for this restoration, but that is not enough. It will require THE FASTING PRAYER TO SEE THE GIFTS MANIFEST THEMSELVES AGAIN. If the early church received them through fasting and prayer, why should we expect to obtain them by doing less than they did? We are more in unbelief now, and faith is far weaker than it ever was before. If anything, it will require more FASTING AND PRAYER THAN EVER before. The gifts of the Spirit will be manifested through fasting and prayer because it is the greatest single agency for spiritual development within the reach and at the command of regenerated man. Jesus is no respecter of persons. When the same factors are gotten together as they were in the Bible, and one has a burden for a specially "coveted" gift, the fasting prayer cannot fail to penetrate through to Jesus to bring the desired results. Failure to do so would be contrary to our Lord Jesus "to profit withal." (1 Cor. 12:7).

Fasting has been a mystery too long for the wellbeing of the human race. This has caused its disuse by the majority, and its abuse by those using it without intelligence. Is it not high time that the value of fasting should be realized, especially in relation to the reception of spiritual power and the gifts of the Spirit?

As members of the Bride of Christ we are like a piano. We are complete in many parts. We are the eighty-eight hammers, the jack hammers, dampers, bridle straps, keys, strings and other parts. Every string of our being and consciousness must be tuned to the pitch of the Spirit. Then the various tones and modulations make up harmony and counter harmony, melody and counter melody. Jesus got His pitch in the consecration fast, and we can get it nowhere else. Spiritually we are "flat," or only tuned in spots here and there upon the eighty-eight note soundboard. We cannot serve as instruments of the higher harmonies unless we fit into our places of the octave of the nine gifts of the Holy Spirit. We first become tuned to the pitch of Jesus Christ in the same manner as He did, by THE FASTING PRAYER.

As well as having Jesus foremost, with our thought focused on Him in the fast, our secondary object should be a burden for the gift we are seeking. It might be a burden for the salvation of souls, or some other objective. Anyway, let us form a triangle out of (1.) JESUS, (2.) the burden we are fasting for, and (3.) self. These three pivotal triangular points must have proper emphasis and contact in the fast. The natural senses diminish and relax, and finally undo the grip of the faster on his natural environment and of the environment on him. The steady focus of spiritual vision on the triangular points blazes into heat and intensity, and consciousness of the natural environment is continually dulled by this double process. The increasing awareness of spiritual environment goes on unhindered and unhampered in the fast, adjusting with great intensity the focus of every faculty on each of the triangular phases. It is like a live wire running from ourself to Jesus, and from Jesus to our need or the gift of the Spirit, and from the gift of the Spirit back to us. When this condition is reached all the way around the divine triangle, our prayer is heard and the gift received. When we look at it with self at the bottom point of the triangle, Jesus at the top left, and our need at the top right, a sacred powerful cross (or atomic circle) is formed, and we know that Jesus hears our cries. Our environment in the natural becomes neutralized and we are attracted to spiritual heights and power to the manifestation and operation of the Spirit. Can this be more plain and logical?

Surely the Lord's people in the near future will put these heretofore hidden secrets of the prophets, apostles and disciples into operation, and there will be a revival of power, gifts in the church, with signs and miracles following.

The Holy Spirit is easily grieved away. When Jesus bestows gifts upon a person through the Holy Spirit, it is very easy for him to lose the gift by grieving the Holy Spirit in failing to live a fasted consecrated life.

I know of different ones who did fast, pray and who received one or more precious gifts of the Spirit. They failed to keep up the work of consecration and fasting, and the Holy Spirit, being even more sensitive after the gifts were received, was grieved and more or less withdrew Himself along with His gift. The gift was no longer manifested. In other words, the line is drawn more narrowly toward perfection, refinement and purity when it comes to the pouring out of His gifts by the precious sensitive Holy Spirit. We believe as the saints of God eventually learn more and more how to go into the complete (forty-day) protracted fast, applying consecration and prayer, there will come in the near future such perfection and refinement that churches everywhere will have completely restored to them all of the nine gifts of the Spirit, "administrations" and "operations." The author feels this is in the making now, and just before Jesus returns, He will have pillars who will allow His Spirit full right of way.

THE REFINERY

As soon as food abstention begins, the blood and energies that have been occupied in digestion, assimilation, and elimination, disengage themselves as such and direct their attentions to something else. The entire body turns into a refinery. A refinery to purify the temple of the Holy Spirit and to purify the blood. The blood will continue for days to be like the crude natural oil that is taken from the well—heavy, dull, and dark in color. The blood goes throughout the whole body in a process of refinement.

REFINING FIRE OF FASTING

IN THE STATE OF RECEIVING A GIFT

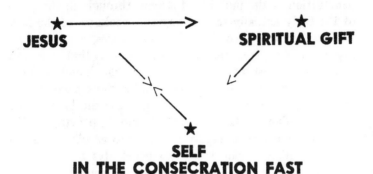

★ ─────────> ★
JESUS   SPIRITUAL GIFT

★
SELF
IN THE CONSECRATION FAST

After the focusing of our consciousness on Jesus and object

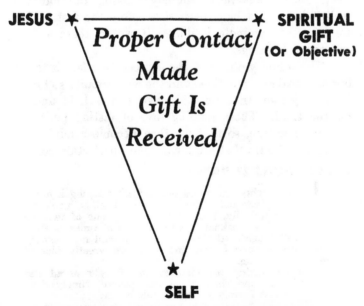

JESUS ★ ───────────── ★ SPIRITUAL
GIFT
(Or Objective)

Proper Contact
Made
Gift Is
Received

★
SELF
AFTER THE PROPHET'S LENGTH FAST

The very weakness that is felt in fasting is a sign this refining process is going on and on. Finally the blood becomes thinner, purer, and highly refined, until it can go through all the blood vessels, even hair-like ones. This penetration of the pure blood stream through all the parts of the body actually takes away the weakness of the fast. Even at eight or ten days, in many cases, a person will begin to feel stronger, and will retain that strength throughout most of the fast. Where the blood is more poisonous and the refining process takes more time, it may require two or three weeks of the fast for the blood to be entirely refined. Highly refined blood penetrates the farthest. When oil is highly refined into gasoline or kerosene, this highly refined oil also penetrates farther.

One can make this test. Place a drop of crude oil on a cloth and notice how far it penetrates. After refinement a drop of kerosene or gasoline will penetrate all through the cloth. Fasting will do exactly the same thing to the blood. It causes it to become so pure that it goes through all the blood vessels and penetrates places where even disease has been, thereby making the individual well if he should have been sick before the fast. Therefore, fastings promote healing. However, these are only secondary blessings.

The primary object in the consecration fast is to have our spiritual nature refined and the old carnality so brought into subjection that we will have a new hold and grip on the Lord. These refining fires of fasting purify and purge our nature, so that we then become candidates for the spiritual gifts that are for us when perfection comes.

MAN 81 FASTS 21 DAYS

"I am eighty-one years old and after trying a number of short fasts and finding them beneficial, both spiritually and physically, I undertook a long one of twenty-one days. The weakness became severe at times as Brother Hall taught. At times I felt fine, and my memory gradually became better, and the Lord greatly blessed me while fasting.

"After fasting, my memory was fully restored and the stiffness and rheumatism disappeared. Ninety days after the fast I can say I never felt better.

George Anderson," San Diego, Calif.

TAKING A FORTY DAY FAST

"AND WHEN HE HAD FASTED FORTY DAYS AND FORTY NIGHTS HE WAS AFTERWARD AN HUNGRED." Matt. 4:2.

There is NO GREATER SCIENTIFIC DECLARATION IN THE WHOLE BIBLE THAN THE ABOVE PASSAGE OF SCRIPTURE.

Practically all medical men and health authorities agree that when a man, woman or child has real hunger for food it is a certain indication of good health.

The fact that Jesus was "an hungred" indicates Jesus took a natural fast as you or I would do. It is a sad fact that some well-known commentators and copyists have interpreted the fast of Jesus as miraculous, and declare that only Jesus could have fasted for forty days. It is possible for practically any adult TO FAST FORTY DAYS, FEEL YOUNG, AND HAVE TREMENDOUS POWER WITH GOD.

Why fast forty days? Is a forty-day fast like a forty-day time clock that opens at the end of a certain period?

To a person who has never fasted or heard of fasting before, "forty days" may seem a long time to fast. However most people can fast much longer than forty days without any harm.

In Christ's time, after a fast was taken by the average person, he would become hungry around the end of a forty-day period. Today the average individual is OVERCHARGED WITH SURFEITING," Luke 21:34, to such an extent that very often it will take longer than forty days of fasting for true hunger to return. This is a sad state of affairs for Christian people to be in, but it is nevertheless true. This explains why faith and the power of God are crowded out. Jesus said men would be "eating and drinking" when the Son of man came.

When a person gets along in his fast as far as twenty some days, it is not much more difficult to go on to his fortieth day. Spiritually speaking, there is a certain ZONE that one gets into about this time (after the body becomes cleansed) that is actually incomparable with any other stage of fasting. When all of the factors are gotten together and our members and consciousness are centered on JESUS in the FAST, the prayer and FASTING PRAYER become more and more penetrating and a GREAT DYNAMIC CLIMAX IS REACHED. This is usually reached between the thirty-fifth and forty-fifth day of the fast. It could, in some instances, be sooner or it could be later. It is like drilling for oil. A certain depth is reached hour by hour, day by day, and week by week. All of the time a little more headway is being made, inch by inch, foot by foot, until finally the pay stratum is reached and a great gusher of oil comes forth. That is the way with a forty day fast. GOD CAN CERTAINLY BE REACHED. He is within our grasp, but we will have to go far enough to make the contact. There may be some misunderstanding here. Some will say, "I reached God when I got saved, or when I prayed through I got victory and reached our Lord." This is true, but I am speaking of a more intimate closeness to Jesus. A closeness as though you are standing in the very presence of His Majesty; a nearness that overshadows the time you were saved and even the time you received the Holy Spirit. Your capacity will be enlarged. Instead of a thimble-size experience, you now will have a bushel or well-size capacity. It will be a bigger experience than when you were Baptized in the Spirit. Nothing pleases the Holy Spirit better than for us to get real close to Jesus, and this closeness is fully realized in a forty day fast. It is the power experience of Luke 24:49.

The display of power and super-manifestation that can be reached on the forty-day time scale of fasting is within the finger-tips of us all.

It is for the rich, the poor, the high and low. It is extremely economical. Practically no one can find a reasonable excuse why they should not take advantage of such a highly beneficial experience sometime in their life. Let us all get started on a very good thing whether we fast only one week or forty days. After we get started in the "FASTING" practice, we will fast more often and the more we practice *fasting through,* the more we will have from the Lord and the longer we will live. Some health experts state that the average individual who eats properly and takes a series of fasts regularly can add from twenty to thirty-five years to his life.

Let us not be guilty of committing suicide twenty or more years before our work is done just by failing to FAST and eat right. The older one is, the more he should fast.

FASTING AND STARVATION ARE TWO DIFFERENT THINGS

It is physiologically impossible for a person to die from the effects of a consecration fast. Fasting is not starvation as some may be led to believe. Fasting is beneficial and rids the body of disease, while starvation is detrimental, and if continued long enough, ends in death. To eradicate any trace of fear, because one can not accomplish the spiritual good that he intends unless fear is dismissed, I want to say there is a fundamental difference between these two processes, and this distinction should be carefully borne in mind when discussing or considering the fasting prayer.

When true hunger returns after around forty days, more or less, of fasting, starvation begins. It is not physiologically possible for death to occur after starvation sets in until forty to fifty per cent of the body weight has been lost. A consecrated fast is never carried to this extreme, and to the point where one suffers so great loss of weight.

People have been known to die while on a fast, but it was because they were already in a dying condition, or had some serious affliction they were suffering from, and would have died anyway. They chose a fast, or were forced to fast as a last resort, and clung to the fast as a last straw of hope.

The destructive force of fear, the mental and emotional fright people experience at the prospect of starving to death, has caused many a person to die prematurely, with or without food in shipwrecked vessels, mine explosions or like tragedies, even where water was present.

Dr. Linda Burfield Hazzard states in "Fasting for the Cure of Disease" that in all the thousands of cases where fasting has been employed there have been but eighteen deaths reported. Two of these patients were only partially fasting, and in every instance it was definitely determined that there was such organic destruction or developmental deficiency of one or more vital organs that death was inevitable whether or not the fast had been taken. Some of the conditions resulting in death were extremely severe, such as abdominal adhesions, interfering with the activity of the vital organs of elimination, syphilis, destruction of liver or kidneys, brain or lungs, atrophy of some organ, or marked arrested development of the intestines, spleen, bladder, heart, or lungs. It was obvious that no system of treatment of medical man or surgeon could have been helpful.

These deaths could not have resulted from starvation, but from the above-mentioned conditions. It was found that in every case there still was considerable subcutaneous fat, which is always entirely absent where death has resulted from starvation. The heart was also normal in all cases, except where it had never been completely developed. In starvation the heart is always contracted or markedly atrophied. In fasting the blood is practically normal in amount, with no real anemia; while in starvation the blood is reduced and there is definite anemia. The pancreas is little affected in fasting, where in death by starvation this organ has practically disappeared.

When death occurs in fasting it is not due to the utilization of all nutritive material, but is probably due to the failure of some particular vital organ or life process. There will always be someone condemning the fast and if someone does die while on a fast it will be magnified and talked about everywhere. People will die whether on a fast or feed, it makes no difference, but the truth is that every day thousands of individuals die from over-eating and nobody ever thinks it is horrible. If someone goes on a fast and dies, who would have died anyway, the last of it is never heard. There are far more people dying from over-eating than from under-eating. After wearing out one set of teeth, many a person secures another set with which to finish digging himself a grave.

The author has seen thousands of people on a protracted fast but has yet failed to see a person die from fasting. Some have gotten into a "mess" by breaking the fast improperly, others have failed to drink the proper amount of water and drank it too cold, some tried to drink coffee when fasting, and some difficulties were experienced because of a lack of understanding of some very simple facts with which they should have been familiar.

WHY FORTY DAYS?

The number forty has to do with humanity. It is made up of the perfect number of order, ten, and the world number, four, which is sometimes called the number of humanity. Forty has to do with the number of days that it takes for the complete subjugation of the flesh. It stands for the time of testing and preparation for the bigger spiritual things ahead for us. It also symbolizes a greater development of the fruits of the Spirit. Humbleness, pridelessness, meekness, patience and a depth of experience are related to it.

Moses, Elijah, and Christ each fasted forty days. Moses' life of one hundred and twenty years was divided into three forty-year periods. The children of Israel wandered forty years in the wilderness before they were permitted to go into the promised land. Unfortunately they had to learn the hard way. The children of Israel could have been in the promised land in a few weeks, instead of forty years, if they would have learned certain lessons.

It appears that one of the biggest lessons that they should have learned but did not was in relation to their *eating habits*. They could not get their mind and attention away from the land of Egypt, or the world. They remembered too easily the carnal things that were left behind, especially their "leeks, garlic and onions." It was impossible for God to lead them into the land of Caanan directly, as they would not give up those worldly desires, cravings, and appetites for the land of Egypt. There were two ways by which this could have been done. Their environment could have been changed over night, so to speak, through fasting. (Fasting is the greatest and fastest method known to change one's environment). The second method was the long way—let them go through a continual grind for forty years in order that their stiffneckedness, stubbornness, and rebellious spirit might be broken. The latter was not God's directive will but it was forced upon Him. "Not for thy righteousness, or the uprightness of thine heart, dost thou go to possess their land." Deut. 9:5. Conditions could have been changed so they could have been in the promised land, perhaps in **forty**

days instead of forty years, if they would have yielded
obediently to the Lord from the beginning. God actually
had to put the Israelites on a forced fast, and they mur-
mured and complained about it. If they had only BE-
LIEVED that God's ways were better than man's ways
they could have had much more enjoyment and saved
themselves a lot of suffering. These are lessons for us to
remember in our Christian experiences. "When thou shalt
have eaten and be full; Then beware lest thou forget the
Lord, which brought thee forth out of the land of Egypt,
from the house of bondage." Deut. 6:11, 12. The Israelites
would not let up and forget the Egyptian false desires
and pleasures. God could not take them into the land of
promise while their affections were still in the world. They
would have to become detached and "unfastened" before
they could expect to enjoy another country. This same
thing applies to the Christian now. Before we are ready for
Heaven, we will have to unloose ourselves from all world-
liness.

To make it easier for His people God put them on a
forced fast. Deut. 8:3: "He humbled thee, and *suffered thee
to hunger,* and fed thee with manna, which thou knewest
not, neither did thy fathers know; that HE MIGHT MAKE
THEE KNOW THAT MAN DOTH NOT LIVE BY
BREAD ONLY, BUT BY EVERY WORD THAT PRO-
CEEDETH OUT OF THE LORD DOTH MAN LIVE."
(See Matt. 4:4) This is the same scripture that Jesus
quoted to Satan at the conclusion of His forty-day fast.
Jesus must have been studying the history of the children
of Israel before He fasted forty days. Even Jesus, at the
age of thirty years, must have seen the necessity of going on
a forty-day fast before He began His ministry. His observations of the many failures of the children of Israel,
their complaining about food, their lusting after eating,
(Deut. Ch. 12), their many murmurings, must have
implanted in His soul a realization of the necessity of accomplishing in a victorious manner what they could not
do. Jesus was more than a conqueror because of FASTING
FORTY DAYS. The children of Israel were defeated because they did not have complete victory over the flesh.
They failed to accept the chastening of God.

A picture of the condition of Israel is brought to us
more vividly in Psalm 78: verses 18, 25, 29-34: "They

tempted God in their heart by asking meat for their lust.—
Man did eat angels' food: he sent them meat to the full.—
They did eat, and were filled: for HE GAVE THEM
THEIR OWN DESIRE; They were not estranged from
their lust. But while their meat was yet in their mouths, the
wrath of God came upon them and slew the fattest of
them, and smote down the chosen men of Israel. For all this
they sinned still, and believed not." Their appetites were
not surrendered to God. They did not "LIVE BY EVERY
WORD THAT PROCEEDETH OUT OF THE MOUTH
OF GOD." To do this it would absolutely require fasting. To "HUNGER AND THIRST AFTER RIGHT-
EOUSNESS," one must get off the eating habit and become empty enough and hungry enough to permit the
spiritual appetite to become properly developed.

Fasting will be a method of self-chastisement and will
prevent numerous sufferings, complications, accidents, and
much other forced discipline from the hand of God. It is far
better, regardless of the many trials and the necessary
will-power brought into play during the fast, to volun-
teer with our free will to subjugate the flesh through food
abstention, whether it be for a few days or forty days,
than to have to come under the severe chastening of the
Lord which may be far more trying. If God's children will
keep their bodies under they may escape much of the
suffering Israel was called upon to endure.

The will-power is tried very severely until after hunger
leaves which is a few days after the fast is started. Even
then one will be confronted with habit hunger. The individual, after the first several days, will be in a condition
of lassitude or weakness for perhaps ten or more days. Dis-
couragement and sometimes despair will manifest itself.
The misery of fasting begins, which is victory over the
flesh. There is no time to let up, because the fast is truly
a fight, and victory is certain if one never lets down.

The sensations of habit hunger cause the stomach
to move about. This is known as peristaltic action, and it
subsides frequently only to appear again, probably around
the next meal-time. This should cause no alarm, although it
may be very painful at times. Sometimes drinking cold
water instead of hot or warm water will aggravate the
condition. Many times pains or cramps will be felt in the
muscles. This is just a normal condition, and a sign that

the poisons are working loose in the body. Your headaches and weaknesses are nothing more than the oxyda-
tion of unassimilated materials that are being consumed.
Sometimes even a fever and other symptoms may show
up to try one, and the many imaginings about the harm
of the fast must absolutely be abolished. We cannot get
things from God when fearful. Please remember the fast
cannot hurt you, but if not broken properly and with
temperance, harm could come afterward. It requires just
as long a period of breaking in and becoming adjusted to
food as the length of the fast. Please remember this.

Many times after one has fasted ten or fifteen days
some natural physiological manifestation shows up that
may scare the candidate into breaking his fast before he
has actually "FASTED THROUGH" on the subject of
prayer. Later he will realize that it was only Satan dis-
couraging, and he will regret breaking the fast.

If a three-day fast is helpful in getting results, why
would not a seven-day fast be more helpful for greater
things? If a seven-day fast is good, a ten or fourteen-day
fast will be even better. If a fourteen or twenty-one day
fast is more beneficial, then a forty-day fast, under some
conditions, should be tops in our Christian experience.

Great spiritual battles may be fought at certain in-
tervals in a long fast. You may have one at fourteen or
twenty-one days and receive great victory, only to find
some more of them off and on along the forty-day trail.

THE BIG FIGHT

Even then you are not through your fast and the greater ac-
complishments can only be realized and brought to maturity after
you have the big fight that is awaiting you in the fast. Finally
a great big one is entered into, or maybe it is in this one major
battle that you will have before the "fast through" VICTORY EX-
PERIENCE. This big spiritual fight, which will be the greatest
spiritual battle of your entire Christian life, usually comes from
the thirtieth to the fortieth day, sometimes after forty days of
FASTING. Herein lies the whole secret of the success of the
fast. You have at last mastered a situation similar to the one that
Christ mastered after "HE WAS AN HUNGRED."

The success is the "FAITH THAT WILL REMOVE MOUN-
TAINS," AND POWER THAT YOU NEVER DREAMED OF HAV-
ING BEFORE. DEMONS ARE AT YOUR COMMAND. You can pray
prayers at a distance and have them heard easier than you could
get results before the extended fast by laying hands on the person

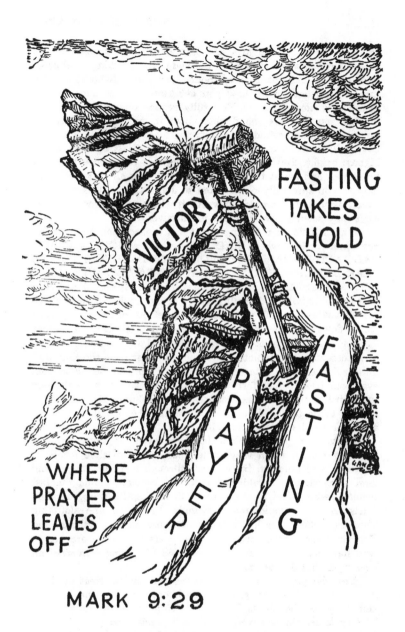

FASTING
TAKES
HOLD

WHERE
PRAYER
LEAVES
OFF

MARK 9:29

FASTING POWER

We believe Jesus' teachings. He taught us there is more power in fasting and prayer than in prayer alone. If our prayers are not answered, then we have access to the greater power of fasting. By fasting and praying to Jesus, the promise is certain. Why live a defeated life?

right before you. The joys and glories are unspeakable at this time; your spirit wants to leave the body; you do things that seem unbelievable and unsurpassed. Sometimes you will be at a place that you do not realize how you got there. A new super manifestation is now available. You fully realize how much of a son of God you now are, no doubts about it, no mistaken identity, no pussy-footing around, no doubts any more to confront you. You have fully reached the depth and you have at last attained to the highest height. You have plowed through an experience that will be so rich and sweet that it will stay with you all of your life as long as you stay fully consecrated to Jesus Christ. This ought to sound as though it would be worth it whatever the cost. Strange as it may seem the cost is not prohibitive.

What I have been talking about is a consecration fast of forty days, more or less, where the Christian wants a FIGHT, a SPIRITUAL BATTLE AGAINST THE FORCES OF DARKNESS. PLEASE BEAR IN MIND THAT THIS KIND OF FAST CAN ONLY BE ACCOMPLISHED BY HOURS OF PRAYER EVERY DAY. The first few days will be difficult because of the weakness, but believe me, that weakness will wear down and get out of the way just as the shadows of the night crawl away as soon as the dawn of another day comes forth. That is why a fast of several days cannot be nearly as successful as a complete fast, which is a fast from the time that hunger leaves until hunger returns. This kind of fast is seldom ever completed before forty days. It is necessary to pray through the weird, dark, trying experiences and absolutely get VICTORY. Failure to do this will result in the FAST being fruitless so far as major results are concerned.

I have seen people go into fasts and even fast several weeks, but they fainted when they came upon those invisible forces of darkness, and failed to battle them through in much prayer and then some skeptic would make critical remarks about the fast being a failure. Sad to say most of these skeptics were so-called Christians but would more fittingly be called the doubting Thomases who never had a word of praise about anything from God since they were saved so many years ago. They are people who have let it leak out and have need of getting converted all over again but do not know it.

Yes, the powers of the evil forces will be so great at times it will take all of the grit and backbone and stamina one has and the grace that Jesus Christ gives to go through and win out. Victory is certain however, if one will persist and press into the fast with all the might and strength he has. The cost is little as compared to the rich rewards that stand in store for one who will be victorious. Let's be a Daniel, an Elijah, a Moses, a David or a Paul, when it comes to fasting. Let's go after it. To be like a prophet, take a prophet's-length fast.

ELIJAH'S FAST

Elijah was one of the most spiritual men that ever walked the face of the earth, and from a study of his life it appears he fasted often in addition to his forty-day fast. John the Baptist fasted often and is a type of Elijah. At one time Elijah ate so little that an angel was sent to him with food. Elijah had been accustomed to eating so little that it appears he was not allowed a heavy meal at one time, but food was given to him in installments so he would not become ill by the over-use of it all at once. "He did eat and drink, and laid him down again." I Kings 19: 6, 7, 8. Again the Angel of the Lord came "The second time, and touched him, and said, Arise and eat; because the journey is too great for thee. And he arose, and did eat and drink, and went in the strength of that MEAT (food) forty days and forty nights unto Horeb the mount of God." Famines did not worry Elijah, he trusted in the Lord and the Lord sent birds, widows and angels to feed him.

It is very evident that Elijah had been fasting before he ate when the angel came to remind him to eat. After his prayer for God to send fire upon the altar during the contest with the prophets of Baal, he told Ahab, "Get thee up, eat and drink; for there is a sound of abundance of rain. So Ahab went up to eat and drink. And ELIJAH WENT UP TO THE TOP OF CARMEL; and HE CAST HIMSELF DOWN UPON THE EARTH, AND PUT HIS FACE BETWEEN HIS KNEES, and said to his servant, Go up now, look toward the sea. And he went up and looked, and said, Go again seven times." —"There was a great rain." 1 Kings 18: 41-45. Elijah, on a fast, out ran Ahab on a full stomach. (Vs. 46.)

A close study indicates Elijah had been fasting even before he went on his forty-day fast. While he told Ahab to go and eat, there is no mention of Elijah's eating. He was too much concerned with praying for FIRE to come down from heaven, and with the destruction of the false prophets, and to praying through for the rain he knew God would send. Elijah had been warned that Jezebel was going to slay him for destroying her four-hundred-fifty false prophets, so he had to flee for his life, still without food. Elijah had been under a very great strain and won a spiritual battle, as it were against hell itself. There was a famine in the land and Elijah was to be the man through whom God would work to correct the condition. He met only stiff opposition from Ahab, and then the false prophets were in his way. Surely he must have fasted to come through all of the tests so victoriously. At the conclusion of all his great victories, he was so wrought up over the fact there were so many false prophets, and so few of the Lord's prophets, and with Jezebel after him he became so discouraged he wanted to lie down and die. 1 Kings 19:4.

"He went in the strength of that meat forty days unto Horeb the mount of God." Elijah was active during his forty-day fast; he took a journey. "He went." Elijah well understood fasting, and he was not afraid of it. He knew that a person obtained more from God when fasting than when he had a full stomach.

We have been studying how fasting made a prophet famous. Your attention is directed to some present day fasts.

Here is the testimony of a brother who fasted twenty-seven days and five sinners were definitely converted in answer to his fast. Did this fast pay off?

"I praise Jesus for giving me the light on fasting through the book "Atomic Power With God", which so ably sets forth the scriptural teaching on the subject.

I prayed and fasted for twenty-seven days, without any food. I did not find fasting too difficult. I worked every day, so naturally I did not secure all of the benefits from the fast that I could have received if I had prayed more. The results, however, were very wonderful. I fasted for some sinner friends and relatives, and all five that I was burdened for became saved, some during my fast and others afterwards. If only one got saved, I would realize it was more than worthwhile to fast twenty-seven days. After the fast was broken properly, I felt better both spiritually and physically than I have felt for more than ten years. Fasting is truly a great experience. I recommend it to all."

Your Brother in Christ,
Brother C. R.
Tacoma, Washington.

A FORTY-FOUR DAY FAST

"My first fast lasted seventeen days, and it was not too difficult to fast. I received wonderful physical results, but I was occupied so much with company that I did not receive all the spiritual results that I should have received. I later went into the fast with consecration to the Lord. I fasted forty-four days, I had visions of Christ, and once He laid His hand on my shoulder. He told me to pray for the lost and the sick. I also saw a very beautiful tree, it must have been the tree of life.

I got along nicely in the fast and after the fast was broken carefully, I felt better than at any time in my life.

A sick person that I was led to pray for was instantly healed."

Sister V. D.

San Diego, California

RECEIVED THE BAPTISM OF THE HOLY SPIRIT
WHILE STUDYING FASTING

"Dear Brother Hall:

I received your book, "Atomic Power With God Through Fasting and Prayer" and several of your very interesting tracts. While I was studying your book and the Bible on FASTING, the POWER OF THE LORD CAME OVER ME IN BLESSINGS AND I RECEIVED THE HOLY GHOST BAPTISM. The Spirit just took control of my tongue and body.

This made me realize more than ever that we are NOT DOING ALL THAT THE LORD WANTS US TO DO. If we fail to fast, it is just like failing to pray. We lose out on many great blessings.

The study of fasting has proved so wonderful that words cannot express how thankful I am for this great truth.

May our Heavenly Father continue to bless you in your work, and MAY IT SPREAD THROUGHOUT THE WORLD, causing all who will to get ready for the coming of Jesus.

Thank you,

Mrs. O. W."

Oakland, California

FASTING HAS CHANGED MY LIFE

"Dear Brother in Christ:

I have received your book on fasting and prayer. After reading it, I truly think it is the most wonderful book I have ever read on the subject. My life has been radically changed. I was convicted of being a SURFEITER. (Luke 21:34). I didn't realize that over-eating kept one from having their prayers answered before. Since I have improved my eating habits and fasted, I have had many more prayers answered. I feel the sweet presence of the Lord ever so much closer than before.

I am convinced that I can be of much greater service to Him we love the best by fasting more often. Please send me some more books and tracts so that I can enlighten others.

Mrs. M. S."

Conway, Pa.

PERSONAL TESTIMONY OF SISTER MARY SOMMERVILLE WHO FASTED AND PRAYED SIXTY-TWO DAYS.

"I was born Feb. 20, 1892 in PAOLA, Kansas. My husband,

THE TESTIMONY OF A SISTER
"IN FASTINGS OFTEN"

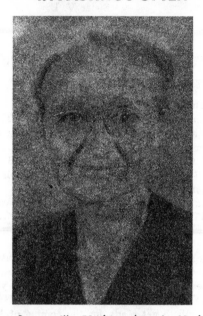

Sister Mary Sommerville 52 days along in 83 days of fasting.

"I HAVE BEEN EXPERIENCING THE GLORIES OF HEAVEN"

"IT SEEMED TOO GOOD TO BE TRUE"

John Sommerville, died twenty-four years ago. I am now living in San Diego, Calif. with my two sons.

"I was not hungry from the beginning of the fast although I cooked three meals a day for my two sons and did all of the housework and the laundry throughout the entire fast. Sometimes I got tired from the lack of rest just like I would get tired when not fasting. I got along nicely and the weakness left after the first two weeks. I prayed four to eight hours a day and attended church regularly as well as being very active throughout the entire fast.

"About two weeks along in the fast I had Spiritual battles, then I saw a vision of 'LIGHT' IN HEAVEN. I gained new victorious ground just after the weakness left me.

"About the thirtieth day of the FAST I became discouraged again and was about ready to give it up. Spiritual powers of darkness were around on all sides. Rev. Franklin Hall came over to my home and gave me new encouragement. He assured me that this was only the work of Satan and great victory lay ahead for me. With this encouragement I continued the Fast and on the thirty-fifth day of the fast the break came. *From that time* on the unspeakable glories of Heaven were all around me in such a way that I wanted to leave this life. I felt like I was sailing all the time, from then on. I felt so light and lifted up. I felt like it would be impossible to stay on earth. I believe that my spirit was carried away at times.

"I went to North Hollywood, to the big tent almost within sight of the 'Universal Pictures.' I had been on the platform shouting and dancing in the Spirit; the next thing I knew I was off the big platform with my hands on a sick person who was in a wheel chair, and the Lord healed her. This was on my 52nd day of the fast. How I got there I do not know. I was told that I had more energy and was more active than any one that was eating.

"It was so wonderful I never wanted to eat again. The experience was heavenly. If Heaven is any more wonderful, I could not stand it. It would be impossible for words to express it. It is an experience that one should undergo for himself. At times I did not want to see or be with anyone, but Jesus. Fasting is a hidden truth but we can all discover it, Thank God.

"The short fasts of two or three days that I have previously taken are no fast at all compared to a long one. You can't possibly understand what a long fast can bring until you pray through those powers of darkness and fast around forty days or more. From the thirty-fifth day upwards through the fortieth day, through the forty-fifth day, through the fiftieth day, through the fifty-fifth day and on through the sixty-second day. Day after day the ecstasy of Heaven, the joy of Jesus Christ was so real. All the thrills of my past lifetime was a bunch of rubble compared to this experience. The experience of receiving the baptism of the Holy Spirit, although precious, is still not to be compared with the joy and power in refillings that can be manifested by the Holy Spirit through a forty day or more fasting experience. I just felt like I was going up all the time and was as light as a feather.

"The strange thing about the fast was I grew stronger day by day."

(Signed) Mrs. Mary Sommerville
2585 Nye Street
San Diego 11, Calif.

SISTER SOMMERVILLE'S ADDITIONAL FASTS

"After fasting for sixty-two days and breaking the fast on diluted tomato and grapefruit juices, I became grieved because hunger had not returned and I believed that I should have fasted longer. After eight days on small amounts of juices, I continued fasting and praying for sinners. Many times I saw visions and had revelations. For many days I felt so wonderful and it seemed that my Lord was right out where I could touch Him. In about twenty-one days natural hunger returned and I proceeded to break the fast. For a week I was on juices, then I went on a milk diet for a few days, and after that into light eating.

"It was not very long until I began other fasts. I would eat about three days a week and fast four.

"During one of the fasts, the Lord spoke to me and told me to go to a certain church the next Sunday morning where I had never gone before. He showed it to me in the Spirit. I got my son to drive me over into the direction where I thought it would be. After about one-half hour of driving we came to a small mission-like church in a thickly settled residential district. I asked my son to stop because this was what I had seen from the Lord. I entered the church and after the preacher got through preaching, I saw a lady in a wheel chair. Immediately I began to rejoice because I knew why I was there. The Lord led me to go over to the afflicted sister and lay hands on her. Immediately the Lord touched her body and she raised up and walked away from the wheel chair, hallelujah! She began walking and shouting. She pushed the wheel chair down the aisle and out in front of the church where the pastor was. The pastor had been taking her home in his car and offered, as usual, to take her home. The healed lady said 'No, PRAISE JESUS, I am healed, I can walk,' and she started walking home and pushing the wheel chair."

The author contacted this sister sixty days later and she was still healed. She told me that she just got in from the garden where she was hoeing and working. She walks everywhere and was so full of happy smiles because Jesus had healed her.

Sister Sommerville joined our evangelistic party in Tacoma, Washington, where we had a great meeting. Scores were healed and baptized as well as hundreds converted. Why? Because of so many scores of God's people fasting and praying. Sister Sommerville fasted 45 days during the Salem, Oregon and the Tacoma, Washington revival meetings. She had such a burden for souls and for God's power to operate. This was another 45 day fast in addition to her 62 day and her 21 day fasts, all within six months.

"In Fasting Often" is a slogan that deep pillars of the faith use and practice when once they taste and see what a major fast will do. Praise the Lamb of God for a quickening among God's people.

I had a contact with five brothers who had recently *fasted forty days* in Los Angeles. All of them received such great spiritual power with God that they informed me they intended after a while to go on another protracted fast. They told me their experience was very precious.

Chapter IX

SOME FASTING PROBLEMS

To present a more complete study of the subject we shall point out and explain some possible conditions that may arise when fasting. Although we are going to explain many difficulties that can come up in fasting, one must not think that all or necessarily any one of these adverse symptoms will be noticed by any individual when fasting with the exception of headaches, dizziness, bad taste in the mouth, lassitude and weakness. Except for the customary "misery" of fasting, most fasters can carry out a long "finish" fast without any great disturbance from these symptoms.

Many times the bowels are not inclined to move easily when fasting, or shortly afterward. The poisonous waste material causes a sluggish condition of the colon. Regular enemas will soften and wash out this putrefaction.

VOMITING AND BILE

Vomiting sometimes occurs early in a fast, though more often there is a sort of nausea without vomiting. Sometimes it occurs late in the fast, but it is more likely to occur in the beginning and in stout persons rather than slender ones. The filth, poisons and accumulations of waste cause the stomach to attempt to eject same. It is usually caused by some organic obstruction of the intestines, to some liver disorder, or to severe congestion. It could be caused by an unloading of bile from the liver and gall bladder frequently caused by reverse peristalsis, which is a flowing backward of bile into the stomach, rather than down through the intestinal canal through which it should properly pass. Enemas are helpful when this condition occurs.

One should drink freely of hot water—one or two quarts if possible, and when this is expelled the stomach will be cleansed and at ease. The water makes vomitng easier because it give the stomach more to contract upon, and its efforts will be less pronounced; also it will tend

to start the peristalsis of the stomach and intestines in
the normal direction. Hot cloths may also be applied
around the abdomen and back. Fresh air and deep
breathing should help. If water is too difficult to retain,
one may take very hot water sweetened with small amounts
of honey or flavored with lemon, orange juice or with
any other pleasantly flavored ingredient. Sucking ice
cubes may also be helpful.

Sometimes the cries of relatives and critics make it
almost necessary to break the fast (when acute vomiting
persists) and try another some other time. When the
above measures fail and the fast is broken, it is not always
best to break the fast on fruit. Thin oatmeal or barley
gruel slightly salted is best; or gingerale, vichy water,
lemonade, or any other acceptable liquid suitable to the
taste. Though the food be promptly ejected, the taking
of a large amount of pleasantly flavored liquid, as previously suggested, will remedy the situation. If effort
is made to break a fast, and the food is ejected, the fast
may sometimes be continued until natural hunger returns.

INSOMNIA:
(THE AUTOMATIC BLOOD TRANSFUSION)

An over amount of blood has accumulated in the
body by an automatic blood transfusion. An individual
loses approximately a pound of weight a day; the first
material used up is, of course, the least useful, along with
certain fats that are stored up in the body. Out of these
fats the good healthy blood is absorbed into other more
vital parts of the body. Some of this blood gets into the
head, warms it up and causes insomnia. The presence of
this large amount of blood helps to explain also why a
process of healing goes on through fasting. IF, AS THE
BIBLE TELLS US, "THE LIFE OF ALL FLESH IS IN
THE BLOOD," HOW CAN ANY ONE DIE TAKING
A FAST? ? ? One does not consume the blood when fasting, and very little of it is lost in a fast. The blood can
actually fight the disease that is in the body by having
a rest from being occupied with the disposition of food.
The blood itself becomes cleansed by the process, and the
body automatically sets up a blood transfusion from the
less vital parts of the body where the blood has been.

Thus it is apparent that fasting is a natural scientific

procedure and is in accordance with the laws of God. If people were seeking healing from the Lord and fasted and prayed to Him and were not healed in the first part of the fast, God would obligate Himself to heal them miraculously. God's ways are so much superior to man's ways that we should believe Him and obey His words where He tells us "Then SHALL THEY FAST." (Matt. 9:15)

DIFFICULTY IN URINATING:

This is an occurrence that is rare and is usually caused by tremendous amounts of wastes and poisons overloading the kidneys during the first part of the fast. Plenty of hot water drinking and enemas will usually remedy the condition. If this fails to help, a very hot bath with only the abdomen submerged, or a sitz bath will usually bring relief. Sometimes either hot or cold ice packs around the bladder will help. Friction skin rubbing is also helpful.

It is very important to relax and get sufficient rest. It is always wise if your prayer life is not too intensified, to have a nap or rest once or twice a day besides the regular sleep, whether or not any kind of trouble develops. This will be a preventive to any irregularity and will make it easier to concentrate more of your energy into your spiritual life when you do pray.

PAIN IN THE HEART, PALPITATION, ETC.:

This occurs very rarely and usually is caused by gas in the stomach pressing against the heart. Drinking two or three glasses of water will generally relieve this condition; also one should sit or lie down and relax. This condition is only transitory and the disturbance is a minor one.

ABNORMALLY RAPID OR SLOW PULSE:

Occasionally nervous individuals are inclined to have a rapid pulse during the fast, at least more rapid than normal.

A cool or cold bath is one of the best measures for controlling rapid pulse. One should continue in the bath until the pulse is about normal.

For a slow pulse, exercise and hot baths should be taken. However, unless the pulse drops below fifty beats per minute or there is a decided drop in the circulation, indicated by increased coldness of the extremities or a tendency to blueness of the lips, no attention need be given this condition.

WEAKNESS:

While the loss of nervous and muscular energy is weakness, generally a person just feels weak, and when the muscular energy is called upon, the strength is there. This artificial feeling of weakness is only LASSITUDE and must be distinguished from real weakness. Lassitude and weakness are not uncommon symptoms on the fast, though there is considerable variation as to the time they may appear and in their degree. These feelings are customarily felt during the first and second stages of the fast and give way to a feeling of increased strength and energy. Lassitude in particular is likely to disappear; a real weakness may not, but very often it disappears also.

Weakness appears most frequently and noticeably in those cases in which drugs have been used in large quantities in the past, also in those who have used tobacco, coffee and alcohol. In long standing cases of auto-intoxication (over eating) the condition will be present. Generally a person imagines his lassitude is a far worse condition than it is. The best procedure to use in controling these feelings is to move around, gradually increasing your exercise, take walks, breathe fresh air and pray harder. These things work like magic. If the condition is real weakness instead of lassitude, more sleep and rest will alleviate it. When a person is just tired, and confuses this condition with weakness, more relaxation and sleep will provide a remedy,

HUMMING IN THE HEAD:

Quite often this is caused by anemia of the brain, and is usually temporary. The excretion of wax is another method used in eliminating waste from the body and may be one cause for the ringing noises in the head. One could massage the neck about the ears if the condition does not disappear in a few days. This condition is rare, and usually is not of long duration.

Sometimes light flashes and specks appear before the eyes. These also are rare in occurrence and may be caused by a toxic condition of the liver or insufficient elimination through the kidneys or bowels. I am mentioning these conditions to show you what may come up, but in the majority of cases one should just forget about them as they are of minor importance.

HICCOUGH:

This is caused by a spasmodic contraction of the diaphragm and sometimes develops in a long fast. It is usually caused by bile in the stomach, and sometimes by intestinal obstruction. It also is not very important, but if it should continue too long may cause loss of sleep and a weakened condition of the body. The sucking of ice cubes, the inducement to vomit, or a hard tapping of the middle region of the back will be helpful. The tightening of a belt around the waist, gradually increasing the pressure, will also assist in remedying the condition.

BODY ODORS AND FOUL BREATH:

The odors from the skin frequently are different from the normal and are greatly intensified during a fast. This is a good sign of the benefits of the fast. Frequent bathing and extreme cleanliness is encouraged throughout the fast. In time both skin and breath will become as clean and pure as that of a child's. Enemas are helpful in this condition. Jesus said, "Wash thy face." (Matt. 6:17).

Many excuses are given for not fasting because of the bad breath with which one has to contend when working at the altars and around the public. Menthol crystals will solve the problem. A tiny crystal placed on the tongue will be sufficient to sweeten the breath, and will last a long time. A quarter's worth purchased at the drug store will last through many fasts. I am offering this as a suggestion only for those who may be sensitive about their breath.

ETHER-LIKE BREATH:

Sometimes there is an ether-like odor on the breath. This is caused by the presence of acetone, which is present in all body secretions, particularly during a major fast. It is probably caused by a decided functional disorder with a breaking down of organic matter. It is particularly likely to develop in a corpulent individual. It is not an especially favorable symptom, and the protracted fast may prove adverse for the extremely stout. Sometimes it is desirable to break the fast when this symptom develops, although a small amount of fruit juice, vegetable broth, or thin oatmeal gruel may serve to end the condition.

CRAMPS:

Sometimes the faster will experience cramping pains in the bowels. These usually are the result of some inner crisis or of a spasmodic contraction of muscles by oversensitive nerves; possibly long retained fecal content has broken loose from its moorings along the colon; or the production of gas from such long held decomposing bowel content. Sometimes it is the result of drinking injudiciously of cold water. Plenty of drinking water, light kneading of the abdomen from right to left and long walks are helpful.

DIARRHEA:

This is a very infrequent symptom in the fast; the tendency usually is the other way. It should be welcomed as a good accompaniment to the cleansing process. The elimination should be encouraged, and a tepid enema may assist in eradicating some pollution, which is very much to be desired in the housecleaning of the body.

BLOATING AND SWELLING AFTER BREAKING THE FAST:

When an individual attempts breaking the fast too rapidly, or eats the wrong food he may experience a bloating, though it may develop days after a protracted fast. In nearly every case it is caused by rushing food in too rapidly for the stomach and other vital organs to become adjusted. It is very important to begin eating slowly and in the right way after a fast. One cannot be too careful in this matter.

When one has experienced this trouble there is one thing that can be done. Stop eating again, and do not drink any water or very little, if any. Take enemas one or more times daily. In many cases, hot bathing is very helpful. Rest and relax as much as possible. After the bloated condition subsides, break the fast and thirst again properly, making sure to allow plenty of time before taking heavy foods. Sometimes it is best to wait much longer before taking milk or food one may be allergic to. If the fast was more than ten days, break the fast on small quantities of food for each meal for many days. If plenty of patience is exercised with the breaking in process, one should experience no further trouble.

CAUTION:

Unless one has a great deal of faith and persistence, there are several conditions that may be present in an individual for whom a long fast may not be recommended. Wasting diseases require extreme moderation in the use of the fast; however many cases of emaciation and general debility have been cured, and the patients restored to normal weight, health and strength. In tuberculosis, where wasting occurs very quickly, it is difficult to gain the lost weight, and only short fasts are recommended and can be repeated often. Even then, some people have been cured by the long fast but I mention this as a caution.

Unless cancer is in its early stages a long fast is not advisable. However, in later stages of cancer this method offers more hope for reduction of the growth and the prolongation of life, (and a more comfortable life too), than any method known.

Those suffering from pernicious anemia will find it better to go on short fasts.

St. Vitus' Dance is caused by a condition of undernourishment and those suffering from it would not find fasting advisable.

Scurvey and rickets are results of a deficiency in diet, and fasting is not recommended.

The third stage, spinal cord syphilis does not call for a fast.

Curvature of the spine is not helped to any degree by fasting.

Pregnant mothers: A fast a few days before delivery often makes delivery easier. Women who are suffering from toxemia or serious functional disturbance of certain organs may, early in pregnancy, take short fasts without detriment, provided their weight is nearly normal, or above.

Most people are under the mistaken impression that even in disease we must eat to keep up our strength, in spite of the obvious fact that strength at such times is not derived from food.

Infant and childhood diseases will disappear, as a

rule, before they are fully developed, if the fast is given at the initial onset or at the appearance of the first symptoms, if no harmful drugs are administered to afflict and poison the little body. Even measles, scarlet fever, mumps, fevers, diphtheria, croup, septic sore throat, pimples, rash, boils, rheumatism, skin blemished, and infantile paralysis, would respond favorably to some degree, if not completely, to a fast for the elimination of the toxic materials responsible for these diseases.

In America the civilized people are so in the rut of eating that they look upon it as a "must or die" necessity. The groove has become so deep that it is practically impossible to get into a sensitive, receptive atmosphere so as to be able to hear the very gentle voice of the Holy Spirit calling us into the deep spiritual things through fasting.

Spirit-filled Indians, Africans, Chinese, and other converts from the mission fields are more easily led by the Spirit into FASTINGS.

A missionary from the Belgian Congo writes to me from Hampton Park, Bristol, England, informing me that the native Christians have had the truth of FASTING revealed to them by the Holy Spirit and they fast on their own. This missionary, however, has decided to start preaching FASTING and spread the truth further since obtaining some books and literature.

I quote part of another letter from England (Hull, Yorks):

Dear Brother in Christ:
Many of our church members and fellow Christians have been much moved in reading your tracts enclosed in a parcel sent by "The Herald of His Coming," of Los Angeles, Cal. Many are fasting longer than they have ever fasted before. They are obtaining results; this is why I know the Lord will bless folk who fast.

I am so hopeful that you will get agents and distributors in England for your material that is so needed here. Christians are sadly lacking the blessings of fasting and prayer. We are very anxious to live lives that are pleasing to Him. Fasting and prayer will surely do this as they can be a great experience. Please send more material to us here; we are hungry for this great teaching.

                                        Yours in Christ,
                                        Sister M. W.
                                        Hull, York, England.

Chapter X

BREAKING THE FAST

"IF THOU BE THE SON OF GOD COMMAND THAT THESE STONES BE MADE BREAD." Matthew 4:3.

The devil also said, "Yea, hath God said, Ye shall not eat of every tree of the garden?" . . . . "Ye shall not surely die:" . . . . then your eyes shall be opened, and ye shall be as gods, knowing good and evil." Gen. 3:1, 4, 5.

Of course Jesus could have turned these stones into delicious lamb chops or anything else He chose. After a complete fast any person is likely to find that true hunger returns in the same way it did for Jesus.

The cleansing of the tongue, the sweetening of the breath, the return of normal pulse and temperature, the sense of rejuvenation and buoyance, the increased circulation of blood in the surface of the body, and a healthy child-like complexion result when the fast is finished and complete. However, some times only one or two of these indications may be sufficient to suggest breaking the fast.

JESUS' words have more dynamic weight and significance than ever before when we find additional hidden meanings to these glorious and wonderful words: "But Jesus called them unto him, and said, Suffer little children to come unto me, and forbid them not: for of such is the kingdom of God."

In more than one way the fasting candidate in a long fast will become as a little child, not only by obtaining simple child-like faith, but he will have the pure sweet breath of a baby, a pure taste in his mouth, and a rosy complexion as well as a brand new stomach that will have to be broken in just like a small child's stomach.

"Verily I say unto you, Whosoever shall not receive the kingdom of God as a little child shall in no wise enter therein." LUKE 18:16, 17.

When the fast has been carried on satisfactorily to its climax, which is usually not before twenty-one days, and more often forty days, or even longer in many cases, depending upon how heavy the person was at the start of the fast, hunger eventually returns. The spiritual victory is, of course, won in the fast-pray-through experience. Sometimes it is necessary to conclude the fast before true hunger returns. However, the premature breaking of the fast is likely to rob the faster of some of the beneficial physical results of a long period of abstinence from food.

At this stage of the fast, the big problem comes before us—how are we to get our new child-like stomach adjusted to food again?

The Word says, "Feed me with food CONVENIENT FOR ME: LEST I BE FULL, and DENY THEE." Proverbs 30:8,9.

Many persons have fasted and prayed very earnestly and secured marvelous and definite results, only to have the old devil appear and tempt them so terribly that they over-ate at the conclusion of the fast and wrecked their bodies though they did not kill themselves.

Satan appeared before Eve, and persuaded her to eat a food which caused her and the race to DIE. Satan also tempted Christ in this same way. Now there was a great object in his appearance at this crucial time when the desire for food was so very real. There is no appetite stronger than the returning hunger after the cleansing of all parts of the body through the fast. This is the most difficult time of the fast. Self-restraint and will power at this time must be strongly exercised. Satan chose this very time to attack Jesus. His object was to tempt Christ to the extent He would turn the stones into a heavy food, eat it, and destroy Himself. Yes, Satan wanted to kill Him. He failed to destroy Him as a babe, and here was another opportunity to do so. Thank Jesus He knew no sin and right here He over-threw the devil by the Word of God. "Man shall not live by bread ALONE." Matt. 4:4.

A new baby has to go into a breaking-in period also, after it is born. The baby breaks a fast. It has to learn to eat for the first time. The first milk from the mother's breast is thin. At six weeks orange juice diluted with half water is given it.

Our breaking in period is very short compared to that of a baby, but we would do well to learn the stomach is brand new, and it will require very slow and gradual breaking in before it becomes fully adjusted to food again.

Many complications can develop. The only safe way is to take it slowly and easily. The more slowly one regains his weight the better he will be physically. If nervousness develops, or any type of ill effect is noticed, one should remember to retard the breaking in period. It will require the same length of time to break in to regular eating as the duration of the fast. If one fasted twenty-one days, it will require twenty-one days properly and gradually to break into regular eating. Lost weight, which is about a pound a day, will not be regained in twenty-one days, it will take much longer to regain all of it. If overweight before fasting, one would not wish to regain all the weight he lost.

Any machine, while gaining or regaining impetus, must begin slowly and work up gradually to higher pressure and speed as it gains momentum. The same is true of the human body—the more slowly it begins its activity, the better. It will be found that if this rule is followed, particularly in relation to digestive activities, trouble will be avoided in the days immediately following the breaking of the fast and in the days to come. A bloating tendency may occur in individual cases where the weight returns too rapidly. This indicates the fast is being broken too rapidly or wrongly. This may be corrected by fasting without either food or water, taking enemas and bathing in warm or hot water, then breaking the fast all over again.

One will experience no difficulty if the fast is broken judiciously. I am offering some helpful suggestions for the proper breaking of different length FASTS:

AFTER A FAST FROM TWO TO FOUR DAYS:—

First day: Three meals of choice fresh fruit, oranges, grapefruit, tangerines, grapes, apples, peaches, tomatoes, or any other agreeable fruit. Second day: Light vegetable meals. Leave off heavy food for several days.

AFTER A SHORT FAST OF FOUR TO SEVEN DAYS:—

First two days: Three or four meals of choice fresh fruit or tomatoes. A vegetable meal can be eaten in the evening of the second day. Moderate amounts of green salads, vegetables, soups, or milk can be eaten for the next few days.

AFTER FASTING SEVEN DAYS TO TWO WEEKS:—

First day: First two meals of fresh fruit juice in six ounce servings. Third meal, choice of (small quantity) fresh fruit.

Second day: Three or four meals of fresh fruit.

Third day: A half pint of any type of milk at each serving, light soups, or very small finely chewed green salads.

Fourth day: Vegetable meals that are green or leafy or milk or soup. Choose a vegetable diet for as many days as you fasted, gradually increase quantity from small diet. Never piece between meals.

AFTER A FAST FROM TWO TO THREE WEEKS:—

First day: Three meals of fruit juice in four to six ounce servings diluted approximately with equal amount of water.

Second day: Three or four meals of same, somewhat less diluted and in larger quantities.

Third day: Three or four meals of choice fresh fruit.

Fourth day: Fresh fruit, milk diet only, soup, or light green salad.

Fifth day: Light vegetable meals, fruit salad, soup, or milk diet.

Succeeding days: Same as above, but quantity can gradually be increased. Stay with a vegetable diet for as many days as one fasted, then slowly go into regular eating but never eat wrongly as one possibly did before fasting.

Cereal meals may be added after fifth day.

AFTER A FAST OF FROM THREE WEEKS TO FORTY OR MORE DAYS:—

Use same method for breaking the three week fast, except smaller quantities should be eaten

and a much longer period should elapse before
taking up regular eating again.

Meals should be spaced four and one-half hours or
more apart. Tomatoes, ripe melons and berries may be
classified as fruit if agreeable. The longer you stick to vegetable meals immediately after the fast the more benefits
you will derive from the fast. And this applies spiritually
also. The spiritual success cannot always be measured
while fasting, but many glorious experiences of victory
are realized afterwards.

Christ observed the Essenes, the Scribes and Pharisees in the way and manner in which they broke their
fasts.

To break a fast hastily and expect Jesus to forgive us
is acting presumptuously. It is like tempting Him.

On a very short fast, the suffering may be noticed in
the stomach, but on long fasts, sometimes the suffering is
not noticed in the stomach but in some deceitful forms that
may manifest themselves in an unexpected manner. At
times it may not be noticeable until days later.

Here is a testimony of a brother 55 years of age who
fasted thirty-two days and broke the fast fine until his
sixth day:

"I have fasted many times for a few days and when I
heard of Franklin Hall's book, "Atomic Power with God"
telling how to fast for forty days, and have tremendous
power with God, I said to myself that Brother Hall was just
a charlatan and it could not be so. Although I went to the
large tent seating two thousand people in Hollywood,
California, within sight of the Universal Pictures Studios,
I did not purchase the book. When I got home that evening, my landlady, 'Mother Craton' placed a copy in my
hands, and told me to read it. After taking the book to my
room and thinking I might glance through it, I finally
got started reading it and actually did not stop until I had
read the book entirely through. It was too logical to pass
over lightly.

"I went on my fast determined to fast for forty days.
I was underweight, about twenty pounds, and fasted 32
days without food. Only pure water was taken. I was
hungry most of the time on the fast, and also quite weak.

"My friends discouraged me from fasting the full forty

days and I broke the fast eight days before I had intended. (I could have gone the full forty, and later wished I had.)

"I broke the fast according to the 'Fasting Book.' The first two days I took less than a glass of diluted fruit juices four times a day. During the next four days I drank fresh fruit juices in small quantities. Then I made a dreadful mistake. It was all my fault and I know I was to blame. I heated one quart of milk, and got a loaf of freshly baked bread from my landlady, and drank the milk and ate the loaf of bread. I became so miserable I went to bed thinking I was dying. To make matters worse, instead of praying and confessing my sin of intemperance, I took some milk of magnesia. I had people praying for me all around. I went on another fast for three days, and God came to my rescue, and forgave me my sin.

"Although I broke the fast in the wrong way, I retained all or nearly all of the wonderful spiritual benefits that I received. It simply is WONDERFUL.

"A cataract also disappeared from one of my eyes.

"I think everyone should know about this wonderful super experience.

"A brother trying to please the MASTER.

G. P."

Los Angeles, California

The breaking of the fast on juices of citrus fruits for several days until the faster has his stomach adjusted to the next step in breaking the fast, will require the utmost care. We cannot emphasize this too strongly. One could wreck his health or even kill himself by failing to exercise will power in the manner in which he breaks the fast. This is especially true after a long fast.

Where the stomach is ready to receive heavier foods, after the juices and fruits, one should eat "LIVE FOODS." Live foods give life and vitality more quickly than other types of food. Live foods are those which can be eaten uncooked, or in their natural raw state. These foods give life. Cooked foods sustain life, but do not give much life. Many persons are suffering from the want of more LIFE, because they eat dead foods. They have their place, but should not be eaten all of the time. It is preferable to eat a meal mostly of the live foods at one time or a meal mostly of the cooked foods at one time rather than to mix the two.

Much live tissue will be required if the fast was a major one, and this comes most easily from live, natural, wholesome food.

This method of eating is more simple, more natural and more as God intended than any other method of eating. The fast actually prepares one for a change in his eating habits anyway. Live foods consist of all whole grain cereals, dried and fresh fruit, green vegetables, nuts, and milk. These and certain other foods supply health, vitality and life-building elements that help to build up the body rather than to destroy it.

More could be said about food, but it is not our purpose to go into the details of such in this book which is devoted to the great spiritual things of God. On this subject I refer you henceforth to "HEALTH FOOD STORES" which have free pamphlets on the subject which should be helpful. They also will give helpful advice.

Whatever your need, whether financial or spiritual, you can have it supplied by prayer and fasting.

I have been glancing through a new book, *"HOW TO BE A SUCCESSFUL MINISTER," by Brother Theodore Fitch. In this fine book I noticed on page 158 a marvelous testimony of many things received in answer to a twenty-one day fast. (A letter from Brother Fitch tells more).

"Jesus meant exactly what He said, "Nothing shall be impossible unto you . . . by PRAYER AND FASTING." In other words, you can do what you desire to do IF you pay the price. That PRICE is the misery of fasting, but the results are glorious.

For instance: "In my attempt to publish this book," writes Theodore Fitch, "I ran out of funds. A few hours after I finished a twenty-one day fast, I received a registered letter from a man I have never seen. It contained the $500.00 check I had to have to put this book on the press. I also received MANY deep things of a spiritual nature that I could have received in no other way. A few days following I received another $300.00 check. Many persons were also healed in answer to my prayers. I received two very precious gifts of the Holy Spirit."

* "How to be a Successful Minister" can be ordered directly from the author, Evangelist Theodore Fitch, Council Bluffs, Iowa (Price $1.25).

Was it worth a fast of twenty-one days to be able to have an impossibility made possible? This was $500.00 that was necessary to finish a book that young ministers, workers, and everyone who wishes to progress and work more efficiently for our Master, NEEDS. This is a 250 page book of many helps for everyone.

FASTING LOGIC

Doctors usually pay too little attention to the matter of diet. If over-indulgence in food is the cause of toxemia, and if one continues to eat too much food or wrong foods, the toxemia remains no matter how much medicine is taken. Anyway, if the medicine should cure the sickness, *the person has to get well twice before being completely cured.* First, he has to get cured of the disease for which he was taking medicine and second, he has to get cured from the medicine that was given him to make him well of the first sickness. The medicine usually contains so much poison the effects of it have to be removed before a patient becomes well. I am, of course, referring to people who do not trust God for their healing. One does not get rid of poison by putting more poison into his system. How then are we to get rid of the poisons generated by improper foods or too much food if we continue to eat? We cannot. No, the way to get rid of these toxins is to *fast.* The sooner people understand the Holy Spirit likes to have a clean, wholesome tabernacle in which to dwell, the quicker doubts and unbeliefs will disappear.

Many people keep themselves tired and exhausted, with their reserve energy expended, by using up the energy of the body in continual digestive processes which are detrimental. The auto-intoxication which results from this excess of food produces toxemia and a poisoning of the tissues and nerve-cells throughout the body, inducing sluggishness, laziness, and an unnatural feeling of fatigue. The degree to which the body energy revives when food is withheld for some days is astonishing, and clearly shows what a large amount of energy is wasted in the digestion and elimination of quantities of food over and above that which we really require. Excess food acts as dead weight.

Is it any wonder then that God's people are sick, powerless, and without strength to labor and travail for the salvation of souls, faith healings, the gifts of the Spirit, and all that Jesus intended for us to have?

A truth emerges from the above argument. During a fast the energy which was previously utilized in the digestion of food material is now set at liberty, and may be used to cure the body, and to give that which we term "energy." I mean both spiritual and physical energy. A vitally important fact is that during a fast the useless and dead matter is first eliminated, leaving the healthy tissues free to function normally. Dr. Dewey states, "Take away food from a sick man's stomach and you have begun, not to starve the sick man, but the disease." Hippocrates also said, many centuries before, "The more you nourish a diseased body the worse you make it!"

Even machinery is given rest periods, periodical checks and is made to stop occasionally. What about man's stomach? A diseased human body is like a machine out of order. Nothing can be more rational than to bring its digestive activities, and vital processes to a minimum while the process of cure is proceeding. This process of repair is a healthy one, and normally uses considerable of the bodily energies.

One of the greatest of all illusions is that it is possible to "support the strength" of the sick person by giving him food. As a matter of fact it has precisely the reverse effect. It keeps the patient weak and diseased for a longer time, and depletes his energies far more than if food had been withheld entirely. Doubtless millions of Christian lives have been lost just because men and women let themselves become "OVERCHARGED WITH SURFEITING" and failed to FAST and live abstemious lives. (Luke 21:34.) No doubt this is mostly due to ignorance. No wonder God's people are perishing for lack of knowledge! Paul says in this regard "WHOSE END IS DESTRUCTION." (Phil. 3:19).

The Scriptures teach us the life of all flesh is in the blood. I have a report concerning blood that was studied in fasting. The report says: "Senator and Mueller in reporting the results of their experiments with the blood of Cetti and Breithaupt, note an increase in the red blood corpuscles in both subjects . . . . In a later examination of Succi's blood, by Tauszk, the conclusions reached were: (1) After a short period of diminution in the number of red blood corpuscles there was a slight increase; (2) the number of white blood corpuscles decreased as the fast progressed; (3) the number of the mononuclear corpuscles decreased; (4) the number of the eosinophiles and poly-nuclear cells increased, and finally, (5) the alkalinescence of the blood diminished."

In Hereward Carrington's book on "Vitality, Fasting and Nutrition," attention is called to cases of fasting in regard to body temperature. It remains subnormal in most cases throughout the greater part of the fast, but has a distinct tendency to rise to normal when natural hunger returns after the body is cleansed (usually from 21 to 40 days). He also has called attention to the fact that in every case observed by him the temperature decreased a degree or more when the fast was broken and the patient began to eat solid food. One would naturally think this would tend to cause the temperature to rise. The fact that body temperature may be elevated by a therapeutic fast has also been attested by Dr. Rabagliati, who says:

"In point of fact I raised the temperature of a man (who was thin, emaciated and attenuated by constant vomiting for seven years) from 96 degrees F. to 98 degrees F., by advising him to fast thirty-five days."

Were our food the sole source of bodily heat and life in the sense commonly supposed, such a result as body temperature elevation by the fast would be impossible, and these results seem to show us the heat of the body is not directly dependent upon the chemical combustion of the food.

Because saints have gotten their mind, soul and body fixed upon the "HAVE TO HAVE THREE MEALS A DAY" to exist, trust in these natural things of life has gone far to cause the true church of the living God to be without FAITH, POWER, and the gifts of the Spirit.

The reason I am presenting these facts is to show how insignificant food is at times when we should be praying and fasting for thousands of sinners who are right now on their way to hell.

A fasting person may feel cold during a fast, particularly if fasting in damp or cold weather. This feeling of chilliness has nothing to do with the body's actual warmth. In the report of one case the person complained of being cold when the bodily temperature was 97.8 degrees F. (or only about .8 degrees F. below normal), on the twenty third day of a fast, while he did not feel the external tem-

perature as being cold when examination showed the actual
bodily temperature was nearly two degrees F. lower. This
shows that the sensation of cold may have little to do with
the patient's actual temperature as registered by the ther-
mometer, but is caused by the condition of the skin, nervousness, circulation of the blood and other factors.

While in some measure the temperature and pulse in
acute disease may rise and fall together, it is a curious
fact that in fasting there is not this correspondence, the
pulse sometimes running up to one hundred ten or one
hundred twenty beats per minute, while the bodily
temperature was nearly two degrees F. lower. This
may drop far below normal without any corresponding fall
in the temperature being noted. Sometimes the pulse drops
very low, to fifty or even forty beats per minute with no
temperature reduction, or other particular effects. I am
giving this information so persons fasting may not become
alarmed at symptoms of this character if they should arise,
since there is no cause for fear.

The quality of the blood can scarcely fail to be improved rather than impaired by the fast. An actual regen-
eration and housecleaning of the blood may occur. In a
short fast of twelve-days, the red blood cell count has increased from 1,500,000 to 3,200,000; hemoglobin increased
from fifty percent to eighty-five percent, and the number of
white cells declined from an excessively high count to
practically normal.

Carnegie Institute Bulletin No. 203 says "The results
of . . . . studies of fasting are conspicuous rather for the
absence than the presence of striking alterations in the
blood picture.

"In an otherwise normal individual," the Bulletin continues, "whose mental and physical activity is restricted,
the blood as a whole is able to withstand the effects of
complete abstinence from food for a period of at least
thirty-one days (the duration of Levanzin's fast), without displaying any excessive pathological changes."

It is possible for forty percent of the fat and muscles
of the body to be lost without danger to the health. The
decrease in the muscles extends also to the muscle cells,
which become smaller. There is no actual reduction of
muscle cells in a fast of ordinary duration. The muscle
shrinkage is due to reduction in the size of the muscle cells.

The heart muscles lose only about three percent, being
nourished from the less essential tissues of the body. Fasting takes a heavy load from the organs, and gives them
less resistance to overcome in pumping the full volume
of blood around the body-circuit. This easing of the
strain enables the heart to repair its structure and im-
prove its function. For this reason many kinds of both
functional and organic heart afflictions have been benefited
and even cured by the natural process of fasting. Circulation also is noticeably improved.

Certain tests have been made of the strength one has
while fasting. A Succi showed on a dynamometer more
strength of the right and left hands on the twenty-first
day of fasting than in the beginning.

Spiritual strength will also be increased, but one does
not always realize it until after the fast.

ALL PRAYERS ANSWERED

"A group of friends and myself have been earnestly
praying, and fasting many times, for someone to come out
strong with the neglected truth about fasting. We feel
that Brother Hall is an answer to this need. All of us
greatly rejoiced when we got hold of the book 'Atomic
Power with God.'

"We believe those who have the Holy Spirit can know
how to utilize this great power in a mightier manner
through fasting and prayer. Brother Hall's book makes
it so much easier to fast and travail with God for sinners.

"I praise God that in a recent ten-day fast that I went
through, God answered all of my prayers. This included
four souls who were saved, several were baptized in the
Holy Spirit, two people were healed and I also was healed,
and feel better than I have felt in years. I also was
privileged to see the greatest revival I have ever
seen here in Portland with thousands in attendance, while
Brother Franklin Hall and Little David were with us in
these meetings. Many folks were saved and healed.
Hundreds of people started fasting for a national revival.

"I feel better than I have felt for years.

Sister K. D."

Portland, Oregon

Chapter XI

THE TRAVAILING PRAYER

FASTING is a protracted season of prayer. It is the travailing prayer. Whenever any crisis of life is seen to be approaching, we should prepare for it by a season of definite fasting and prayer. Better still, we should be prepared ahead of time because sometimes a crisis comes to us so unexpectedly that we do not have time to go into a fasting prayer to prepare ourselves to meet an immediate emergency.

Christ fasted and prayed not only before the great events and victories of His life, but also after His great achievements and important crises in order to be fully prepared for the next battle.

When He had fed the five-thousand with the five loaves and two fishes, and the multitude desired to take Him and make Him king, having sent them away He went up into the mountain apart to pray, and spent hours there alone in prayer to God. We can not picture Him going hunting while secluded in the mountains. We would naturally conclude that He was in fastings. So He went on from victory to victory. Matt. 14:23: Jno. 6:15.

It is more common for most of us to pray before the great events of life than it is to pray after them, but the latter is as important as the former. If we would fast and pray after the great achievements of life, we might go on to still greater victories; as it is we are often either puffed up or exhausted by the things that we do in the name of the Lord, and we advance no further. Many a man has been endued with power in answer to prayer and thus has wrought great things in the name of the Lord. But when these things are accomplished, instead of going alone with God and continuing in humility and deep prayer, he congratulates himself upon what he has accomplished, becomes puffed up, sits down and takes it easy for a while, and consequently God is obliged to lay him on the shelf. The great things done were not followed

by effacement of self, and by prayer to God, and pride
has come in and the big man has been shorn of his power.
Examples of such tragedy can be seen in certain very
successful evangelists of the past who were mightily used
of God, but today they are in some kind of business for
THEMSELVES.

Many a person seeks and tarries for the Holy Spirit;
hours and hours of praying is done and finally God fills
him with this great power. A few weeks or months pass
and they are further from God than before they received
the Holy Spirit just because they left off their prayer life,
and became self-contented and exalted over what God had
done for them.

Nowadays the great excuse is "I am too busy to *pray*
and to *fast*." No one is ever too busy to live on "THE
WORDS OF GOD." (Matt. 4:4) Jesus Christ was
busier than the busiest people, yet He always saw to it
that HE GAVE A SPECIAL TIME TO PRAYER. When
the throngs were crowding around Him, and there were
people to be healed, and men and women needed the
Gospel preached to them, He would withdraw at such a
time from the multitudes and go into the wilderness to
pray. Luke 5.15, 16: "But so much the more went
abroad the report concerning Him: and great multitudes
came together to hear, and to be healed of their infirmities.
But He withdrew Himself in the deserts and prayed."
(R. V.) It appears that the busier Christ's life was, the
more He prayed. No man could be busier than Christ
was, yet He always had time to pray. In other words, no
person whether king or president, banker or business man,
janitor or servant, ever becomes too busy to pray to his
Creator.

We should never take time for other things of life
such as our work or business, housecleaning, cooking, eating, or any other temporal duty until we first take time
to pray. "Seek ye first the kingdom of God and His
righteousness." Many times our blessed Jesus had no
time to eat (Mark 3:20). Sometimes He had no time for
needed rest and sleep (Mark 6:31,33,46), but He always
took time to pray; and the more the work crowded the
more He prayed.

Many a man mightily used of God has learned this
secret from Christ, and when the work has crowded more

than usual they have set an unusual amount of time apart for prayer. Other men of God, once mighty, have lost their power because they did not learn this secret, and allowed increasing work to crowd out their fasting and prayer life. One of the main things that has crowded out their prayer life, and consequently crowded out the faith that they did have, is the time people allow for the preparation and eating of food. It is impossible to contact God properly with an overfed body. Overeating kills faith. When faith disappears, a person becomes powerless. There are times when we should be empty enough to press on toward God to become saturated with His presence and power, and not allow corruptible things to be in us or around us, or to weaken our relationship with the Lord. All the great men recorded in the Bible received power, performed miracles, and came close to the Lord on an empty stomach.

By all means let these facts rest with us and may we never forget the more the work presses us, the more time must be spent in prayer, whether it is just praying, or fasting and praying. Remember, all time and even *our* time, belongs to the Lord.

Our whole life should be a life of prayer. We should walk in constant communion with God. There should be a constant looking upward of the soul to God. We should walk so habitually in His presence that even when we awake in the night it will be the most natural thing in the world for us to speak to Him in thanksgiving or in petition.

Christ's very life was but a definition of prayer and fasting.

If Jesus the Son of God, needed to fast and pray, how much more do we blood-washed sinners need to do so.

A close study of Christ's life shows us that He was very much concerned about food abstention so He could obtain more of the spiritual meat from above. Even the Son of man found it necessary to fast often.

At times the disciples were puzzled by His refusal to eat with them. They were concerned about the natural things too often and Jesus had to rebuke them for it. "But He said unto them, I have MEAT TO EAT that ye know not of. Therefore said the disciples one to another, Hath any man brought Him ought to eat? Jesus saith unto them, *My meat is to do the will of Him that sent me,* and to FINISH HIS WORK." John 4:32-34.

How happy we should be to know that Jesus too, could receive such glorious spiritual results from FASTING. Surely if Jesus knew the great secret of this kind of prayer, we ought to avail ourselves of the opportunities to obtain what is brought about by it. We are ordinary sinners saved by grace, and if Jesus needed it, how much more do we need the power and results that positively will come about through the FASTING PRAYER experience.

Jesus well knew that to obtain the spiritual food it was necessary to deny Himself the "meat" that was carnal. The best meat is to do the will of the Father. Another place Jesus calls "bread" the "word that proceedeth out of the mouth of God." Matt. 4:4.

Sometimes it is necessary to lay aside the natural appetite of hunger and GO AFTER THE SPIRITUAL things of God by food abstention, if we are really going to secure and obtain the healings and super works of God. The four thousand men besides women and children had to give up all, even food, (some gave it up for three days) in order to be with Jesus to receive everything He had for them. Of course we could not imagine Jesus Christ eating in the midst of His people without feeding them so He must have been fasting at that time also. Jesus showed us the example, and if we are to be like Him, we surely will have to follow. (Matt. 15:32).

We are giving a testimony of a sister who did follow Jesus in FASTINGS. She received HEALING FROM HIM and another person was healed in answer to her FAST.

FASTED SEVENTEEN AND FORTY-THREE DAYS

Mrs. Verna M. Dominguez of 620 E. 4th St., National City, California, has fasted many times with splendid results. She states:

"In the Spring of 1946 I fasted seventeen days. I was healed of all diseases and got along wonderfully. It was necessary to do a lot of traveling while on the fast. I drove from San Diego to San Francisco, and from there to Sacramento. I usually get car sick when eating but I didn't have anything in my system to get sick from so I enjoyed the trip more than usual, except that over-solicitous relatives finally persuaded me to break the fast before I really intended doing so. When I started the fast I did not intend taking the trip, but some things came up unexpectedly. I didn't realize the great spiritual results that I should have received if I had prayed more.

"A few months later I started another protracted fast. This time I prayed much and earnestly sought God to secure spiritual power and a refilling of the Holy Spirit. About the time I started the fast I had laryngitis. I was healed of this condition about the eighth day of the fast. I fasted seventeen days and had a spiritual oppression from the devil. I broke the fast and ate lightly for seven days (I wasn't hungry) but was very sorry that I had given up so readily because I had not received what I wanted from the Lord. I took up the fast again and earnestly sought Him. A friend of mine was very sick. I was led to pray for her about the twenty-first day of the fast and God answered prayer and wonderfully healed her body.

"At times it was difficult but I finally got more victory as I continued fasting. I had several visions of the Lord and of Heaven. I saw many things. I was praying for much people and then I saw Jesus come and lay one hand on my shoulder and one on my head. He was so precious to me. The longer I fasted the more real He became. I also had many revelations. I fasted to the fiftieth day, and except for a week that I ate lightly, I fasted forty-three days.

"The first part of my fast I was bothered with peculiar pains in the abdomen. Some other unpleasantness came up occasionally, but when I took walks and drank plenty of water, rested, and prayed; they soon disappeared. I feel better now than I ever felt in my entire life, and I have had a far greater touch from the Lord than I ever had since receiving the Holy Spirit. I am much deeper and know how to let the Holy Spirit use my life better for His glory. When you once get started fasting you want to fast often. Jesus has been so real to me, and I would like to see other Christians learn how to fast."

DO YOU CONTROL FOOD OR DOES
FOOD CONTROL YOU?

If we cannot fast a week or two now and then I am afraid we are under bondage and a slave to carnality as well as an enemy to Jesus Christ. Philippians 3:17-19. Food has control of us instead of our having control of it. Yes! A week or two of fasting is only a short Bible fast and if we do not have sufficient will power to lay aside natural food to obtain more spiritual meat, we are not worthy to expect God to answer all of our prayers. The results are sadly deficient, and we come so far short of the goal that Christ intended for us to reach that it should put us to shame.

FASTING LIVES ON THE VERY POISONS
THAT ONE WISHES TO ABOLISH

Regardless of the great spiritual results of a week or two of fasting now and then, our earthly tabernacle so greatly needs this fast for cleansing that everyone owes it to himself to take a fast of this kind three or four times a year at the very least. Every woman who has a home always gives it a good going over in the spring. She calls it spring housecleaning. Then she goes over the house from top to bottom several other times during the year. Why not give just as careful consideration to the temple of the Holy Spirit? The cleansing of this temple begins with food abstention.

In the spring, after our heavy winter diet, our bodies are heavily laden with toxic poisons, more than at any other time, and are very much in need of housecleaning to remain well and healthy. At the end of summer, just before cool weather sets in, and as a safety first measure against the wintry colds and for fortitude, is another good time to take a fast. Also in mid-winter a few days food abstention will insure good circulation to the system when exercise is at the minimum, and will fortify the body for the rest of the season against disease.

The Scriptures are far ahead of health authorities and medical science. A close study of the Word of God shows us plainly that the best way to live and please our God is by the plain simple way of eating. Jesus said, "MAN SHALL NOT LIVE BY BREAD ALONE." Matt. 4:4. When man tries to live on bread alone there is a physical backfire, so to speak, as well as an unsatisfactory spiritual condition. Let us believe these simple words, "MAN SHALL NOT LIVE BY BREAD ALONE." Man's diet is far from being complete when food alone is depended upon as the entire source of our living. Jesus was referring to fasting as part of the spiritual diet that is necessary to keep us healthy. I believe that this also meant HEALTH FOR BODY, SOUL, AND SPIRIT. As children of God we cannot LIVE properly without taking into consideration the entire man which includes both the spiritual and physical. In Ecclesiastes 5:17, it tells of the sorrow attached to wrong eating and eating in the darkness, or ingonrantly. "All his days also he eateth in darkness, and he hath much sorrow and wrath with his sickness."

It is very sad that many people stuff just before coming to church and then expect to have enough of faith to get people prayed through to salvation or divine healing. Worse still, many churches are so busy preparing dinners and banquets to stuff on right in the church that it is no wonder Christ stands outside of His Own Church. That is why many places of worship are literally dead so far as the power of God is concerned. "It is better to go to the house of mourning, (or fasting) than to go to the house of feasting: FOR THAT IS THE END OF ALL MEN; and the living will lay it to his heart. Sorrow is better than laughter: for by the sadness of the countenance the heart is made better." Eccl. 7:2,3.

If fasting will aid in ridding the body of waste and cleanse it to a high standard of physical perfection for the Holy Spirit who abides therein, how much more effectively can fasting rid the soul of the DOUBTS AND UNBELIEF THAT have been secluded there for so long a time. Just as surely as we fast and pray our spiritual nature ascends to lofty heights, and climbs over doubts and unbeliefs to reach out for the faith Jesus is so anxious for us to have. It hunts up the Lord, who may seem to have been hidden. No longer will we have a sickness or weakness that needs healing, for FAITH IS THE VICTORY.

The fast will bring on the power to pray the prayer of faith more effectively. The prayer will come forth with a struggle but will be an "EFFECTUAL" prayer. It will be a prayer that will be "FERVENT," a PRAYER THAT WILL MAKE CONTACT WITH JESUS. This is the prayer we want because prayer that will not make contact with God is a useless prayer.

Even during the fast, many times doubt will try to scare us out of praying this real prayer, and we may faint and ask what is the use because we do not always feel like praying.

David sensed the great value of the FASTING PRAYER when he said, "I HUMBLED MY SOUL WITH FASTING; AND MY PRAYER RETURNED INTO MINE OWN BOSOM." Psa. 35:13. A lot of people are too proud for God ever to hear their prayers. Even if those same folk do not feel proud, the facts prove they are proud because they would never humble themselves to fast. Fasting is perhaps the best way to kill the old man of pride. Pride lives on the appetites, and fasting masters the appetites, therefore pride may be eliminated by a person who will fast occasionally for at least a week or more. All of the natural appetites cannot be conquered in less than ten days of FASTING or longer. People will understand what I mean when they try a ten-day fast, and they learn they had a lot more pride than they ever thought possible. A fast will show up a lot of things, and will so master the flesh and get it so subdued for a time that the real GLORY OF THE LORD CAN COME FORTH AND THE FAST-ER CAN TRULY BE A BLESSING TO THE CAUSE OF JESUS.

This is what God can do for a person who will mix much prayer with his fast and put every effort into it so that the greatest amount of good can be gotten from the fast. Here is an account of the seventeen-day fast of Mrs. Jewel Wininger, age 31, height five feet, four and one half inches, weight before fasting, one hundred thirty-eight pounds.

"Before I went on my fast, my daughter Gene was on a short fast the day that she received the Holy Spirit. She was lost in a vision and the glory of God was all around her as she and others were lying under the power for several hours. This was in a fasting prayer revival in Hollywood, within sight of the Universal Picture Studios. It was the last night of the revival where Rev. Franklin Hall had been speaking twice daily. The large tent seated about two thousand people and many had been converted, including myself. Many were healed also. Others had gotten the light on fasting and were fasting as long as forty days.

"Although I did not fast very much in that meeting, after the campaign, I fasted seventeen days. Hunger left me on the third day. ALL WEAKNESS LEFT me when I was seven days along. I lost sixteen pounds, but gained it all back later. I was able to pray all of the time, even part of the night. Jesus was so very close to me. I had revelation after revelation. Some were about how God would bless if His people would only start to fast and pray. Anyway it seemed all of heaven was brought near me and I could hardly stand it any longer in this world. On the sixteenth day it seemed my spirit left my body for about two hours. I was shown by an angel the brim of hell where unbelievers go. I could actually feel the heat. I was burdened for sinners. Other things were shown to me but I was forbidden to utter them.

"The experience was so real throughout the fast it seemed

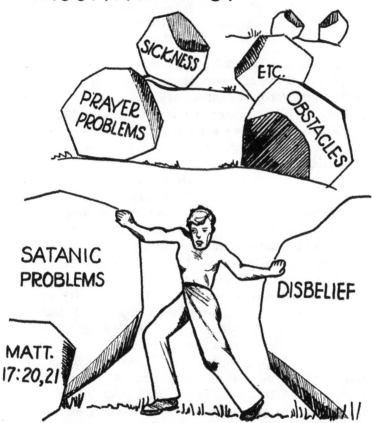

MOUNTAINS OF

SICKNESS

ETC.

PRAYER PROBLEMS

OBSTACLES

SATANIC PROBLEMS

DISBELIEF

MATT. 17:20,21

A CHRISTIAN'S EXPERIENCE WITH FASTING PRAYER

What a prophet's-length fast will do!

that I was under the power all of the seventeen days. I was given a call and burden to preach. I received the precious Holy Spirit the day before I started on the fast.

"It is now a month since I broke the fast and I feel better physically than I have felt in fourteen years. It was so wonderful that I want to be like Paul 'IN FASTINGS OFTEN.'"

Jewel Wininger
5114 Denning,
North Hollywood, Calif.

Fasting is mentioned a great number of times in the Scriptures. There are many places in the Scriptures where fasting and food abstention are indicated along with prayer, or without prayer, but is not called by the name of fasting. However we know that the meaning is similar. Many times Jesus withdrew Himself and went into the mountains, wilderness or desert. We know that He was fasting and praying, although we are not always told that He did pray and fast. Many deep spiritually-minded people have fasted, but it was not their custom to advertise this fast, so we do not fully realize how far the prophets and early church members practiced it.

John the revelator must have been in some long fastings to have received the revelations from our Lord Jesus Christ. The greatness and length of these revelations indicate that John could never have received all that he received, except by intense prayer and fastings. We believe that John, being a devout follower of Christ, observed Matt 9:15. We are not told that he did fast, but from our knowledge of part one of the Revelation, which is the book of Daniel, we believe that John did fast. We know that the prophecies of Daniel were a product of FASTING. Therefore, we can safely conclude that the Apostle John was an experienced faster. John was one of the one-hundred-twenty who we believe fasted in the upper room.

A FASTING HEALING TESTIMONY

Rev. W. H. Guilliams, pastor of the Foursquare Church in Inglewood is a strong advocate of the FASTING PRAYER truth. He preaches sermons on it and practices it with his whole church. His wife just completed a seven-day fast and had some very precious experiences with the Lord.

Brother Guilliams states, "When I was pastoring a church in Colorado a brother of one of my members came to visit him. He was seriously afflicted with dropsy. He was so bloated that as he would walk or move abruptly, one could hear the water moving around in his body. He was much overweight. I became burdened for him and felt led to call my church to fasting and prayer. Without exception every member in the church went to prayer and fasting, and we fasted 'UNTIL' we felt VICTORY for this brother. Within a week from the time we had victory, the person afflicted had lost FORTY-FIVE pounds of weight and was completely delivered and healed. PRAISE JESUS! It has been several years now since this brother was healed and he is still perfectly whole today."

Again Rev. Guilliam relates another fasting case in which a business man was delivered from alcoholism. I quote: "Mr. Frank Tyler Daniels is president of the Daniels Chemical Co. which manufactures the Dozzel cleaners soaps. Mr. Daniels is married to a lady who was pastor of an Assembly of God Church. Mr. Daniels was a very heavy drinker. He drank so much that his wife finally became discouraged, backslid, and gave up her ministry.

"On July 15, Mrs. Daniels succeeded in getting her husband to attend the Foursquare Church where I was pastor. He was drunk when he came into the church. He had been drunk continuously since April 15. This was a period of ninety days. When he came to church he was so polluted with drink that it could be smelled from one aisle to the next. He slipped out to the front of the church and drank the remainder of what he had in a bottle that he had in his pocket.

"He had been to Brother Lee's church and had been prayed for. He had also been to Angelus Temple and was prayed for there. Christians in various places of worship prayed for him but it did not seem to do much good. We felt the burden for both him and his backslidden wife so I asked my church to FAST and pray. When my whole church and I fasted a week, God came on the scene and delivered him from the drink habit, taking it entirely out of his system. His wife also gave her heart to the Lord, and today they are a happy family—made that way through FASTING AND PRAYING TO THE LORD JESUS CHRIST, HALLELUJAH! Several years have passed and when I saw and talked to this converted drunkard recently, he informed me that he had not touched drink from that day to this, and Jesus Christ is blessing him in a wonderful way. He stated that it makes him sick to smell the stuff now."

Rev. Guilliam has seen many miracles come about in answer to fasting and prayer and was able to give many testimonies in regard to this blessed truth. Thank God for a pastor today who is not afraid to come out with this hidden truth, and practices what he preaches.

FASTING PROLONGS LIFE FOR MAN OF EIGHTY-TWO YEARS. FASTED SEVENTEEN DAYS AND WALKED THIRTY-FIVE MILES

"Dear Brother:

Your book on fasting and prayer is very good. I took many fasts in my younger days. I fasted fourteen, ten, seven and two days. One time I fasted twenty-two days. I am now eighty-two years of age. I fasted seventeen days and *walked thirty-five miles without being tired.*

"Thank you very much for the information in the book. What I am concerned about is a Holy Ghost awakening coming to this nation.

"I have found some difficulty in getting my bowels to move while fasting and immediately afterwards, although later on the fasting helps this condition. As a word of advice on long fasts, I suggest that the bowels be cleansed regularly by enemas and during the first of the fast by salt water.

"My difficulty is not so much in fasting as in praying. Holding concentration for one object in mind will go a long ways towards obtaining the BLESSINGS OF JESUS.

"'Although an old man I still intend to fast and keep fasting until I keep growing younger like Moses did.

Brother H. B."
Jackson, Calif.

PASTOR FASTS AND HAS BURDEN LIFTED

"Dear Sir:

Your book came into my hands accidentally. I wish to say that I can accept every bit of it. I received such a blessing by fasting and studying it that the heavy burden that I had carried for many years was lifted. I knew this was God's answer for me. Please mail more tracts and literature on the subject. I want to fast and learn more about the longer fasts so I can teach my church about this great and vitally needed subject.

Pastor H. W."
McCann, Calif.

Chapter XII

DIVINE HEALING THROUGH FASTING AND PRAYER

Matt. 17:21: "THIS KIND goeth not out but by PRAYER AND FASTING." What kind goes out through prayer and fasting? Any kind of sickness or disease that will not respond to prayer alone. No matter what the sickness or affliction may be, and no matter how many demons the patient may be possessed with, Jesus declares if you completely follow His pattern and formula, it can come out. Any thing, within the limits of the will of God can be brought to pass by FASTING and PRAYER.

Sickness and disease are a curse of the law. Sin, sickness, and sorrow are unmistakably identified with the old serpent, the devil. They are the works of Beezlebub. (Mark 3:22). In the twenty-eighth chapter of Deuteronomy, we have explained the curse of the law in regards to disease and sickness. Most diseases are catalogued in this remarkable chapter.

"Christ hath redeemed us from the curse of the law, being made a curse for us: for it is written, CURSED IS EVERY ONE THAT HANGETH ON A TREE." Gal. 3:13. We have healing in the atonement. It is all paid for, praise His NAME! It is a greater miracle for God to save a sinner and wash away his black sins, make him a new creature, and give him eternal life, than it is for Him to heal a sick person. Divine healing or redemption for the body, and eternal life, are like two links in a chain. They are inseparable. How can a person have eternal life without the salvation of his body also? Divine healing is actually a foretaste of the redemption of the body which is to take place later on.

The unholy triplets, sin, sickness, and sorrow, which are the works of the serpent, can be removed through the BLOOD of Jesus. A certain blood remedy was once advertised as, S S S for the blood. This slogan was on bill-

boards all over the country. I believe they have it turned
about. It should be BLOOD for the S S S;—the BLOOD
of Jesus for SIN, SICKNESS, and SORROW. Isa. 53:5:
"He was wounded for our transgressions, He was bruised
for our iniquities: the chastisement of our peace was upon
him; and WITH HIS STRIPES WE ARE HEALED."
This Scripture deals with both healing and salvation in
the atonement. An additional price was paid for our healing. A big Roman soldier dressed as an athlete, took a whip
of nine strips, and pieces of metal were fastened to the
ends of the strips which made up the whip. Jesus was
led to the whipping post; His hands were tied around the
post, and His beautiful back was laid bare. Time after
time His body was lashed and striped. I can see the pieces
of metal as they tear gashes in His back until it was
marred with wounds, and this, my dear friend, was the
additional price that was paid so you might be loosed from
you infirmity, affliction, disease, or sickness. The more
vividly you can picture this scene of redemption for, and
healing of the body, the more quickly you will become
healed. A FASTING AND PRAYER PERIOD WILL
assist one more effectively to get a glimpse of this awful
pre-suffering before Calvary.

"Jesus Christ the same yesterday and today and
forever" Heb. 13:8. Many Scriptures show us that Jesus
is the same, and is as willing to relieve the suffering
TODAY as He was willing to do when He walked the
shores of Galilee. No man has power to revoke, annul, or
repeal these promises and commissions which were given
to all believers. "These signs shall follow them that believe; In my name shall they cast out devils; they shall
speak with new tongues; They shall take up serpents;
and if they drink any deadly thing, it shall not hurt them;
they shall lay hands on the sick, and THEY SHALL
RECOVER." Mark 16:17, 18.

If Jesus did not heal the sick today, He would be a
respecter of persons. He would be an unjust God to heal
folk in His time, and not to heal His people today. We
can not see a righteous God unwilling to heal the afflicted
today.

Mark 16:15-20 is not written in symbolic language,
neither is it written in figurative language, therefore it
must be, and it is written in literal language.

There is not an evangelical orthodox church of any denomination which does not take literally the 15th and 16th verses of the 16th chapter of Mark. They say it is the greatest command and authority for preaching the Gospel in all the world, and it is written, "Go ye into all the world, and preach the Gospel to every creature. He that believeth and is baptized shall be saved. He that believeth not shall be damned." Now, if we take literally the 15 and 16th verses, why not be logical and take the rest of the chapter in the same way?

Jesus said, "These signs shall follow them that believe." He did not say those signs would follow only the apostles, or the early Christians, but "THEM THAT BELIEVE." However, those signs do not follow unbelieving churches and pastors and individuals, but, said the Lord, they follow those who believe—you, me, or anybody else. If you do not believe enough, then fast with your prayers, and YOU SHALL BELIEVE WITH THE FAITH THAT IS NECESSARY.

"In my name shall they cast out demons." A great medical scientist of national reputation said some time ago: "A great deal of insanity is not a physical problem for medical science, but it is a spiritual problem for the church, and if the clergy and church were what it should be, a great many insane people would be delivered from insanity and demonism." All insanity is not demonism, and some of it comes through natural causes,—worry, overwork, injury, result of complication of diseases, and the breaking down of the nervous system through over and improper eating.

If God intended doctors should take the place of faith He would be showing special favor to the rich. The further fact that the rich are often enabled by their wealth to secure the services of famous doctors which the poor cannot afford because of their poverty, leads us to ask if it is logical that a loving God should have provided a better means of healing which would be available to the rich, and not to the poor?

We cannot believe it! No, He has provided for rich and poor alike in His own divine and loving power! However, we must, to obtain this healing, meet every condition to the fulfilment of His promises, and there is a condition to be met in which many are failing, and that is prayer with FASTING. When other means fail, this must get the job done.

If sickness is from God, and is a part of His will for us, then Jesus, the Son of God, was constantly overthrowing the works of God, and running counter to His will by healing the sick—all of them that came to Him when He was on the earth.

WHEN DID GOD INTEND DOCTORS TO TAKE THE PLACE OF FAITH?

So many people seem to be under the impression that in this day the Lord intended for us to depend upon doctors and drugs instead of upon faith. If He intended the doctors to take the place of faith, I might ask which school, for I notice there are many different schools in the medical profession. There is a group which does exactly the opposite of what is advocated by the other group. They say they are right and the others are wrong. These schools keep changing. In a few years from now they may be doing the opposite of what they are doing today. Then I might ask in what year, or just when did the Lord intend us to give up faith and prayer, and substitute doctors and drugs in place of it? It is true Christians sometimes make mistakes and some are overzealous in expounding the truth of Divine Healing, but even in this enlightened age great blunders are constantly being made in the medical profession.

I do not wish to imply the medical profession is sinful, or that the use of drugs is wrong. There are, and always will be, innumerable cases where faith cannot be exercised, and as natural means have a limited value, there is ample room for their employment in these cases: but for the true and obedient child of God, there is the more excellent way which His Word has clearly prescribed, and by which His name will be honored and praised through our believing and trusting in Him.

The man who repudiates Divine Healing is behind the times, and is ignorant of the up-to-date findngs of modern medical science.

At a convention of medical scientists in London, Dr. Theodore Hyslop took a position, which he logically sustained, that for a distressed mind, depressed spirits or mental derangement, the best therapeutic agent known to man is to relax, and get into the habit of prayer to his

God. Dr. Hyslop is an authority on the human brain, and is supposed to know more about it than any other person in the world. He further said, "Prayer is the best remedy he ever discovered for insanity. Prayer will rest the tired mind, quicken our weak bodies, and bring sanity to the crazed brain."

DIVINE HEALING ALWAYS IN THE TRUE CHURCH

John Wesley believed and practiced it. There are more than two score of passages in the Journal of John Wesley which prove he believed and practiced Divine Healings. It was common teaching in old Methodism. On August 15, 1750, after reading a book, John Wesley commented: "The grand reason why the miraculous gifts were so soon withdrawn was not only that faith were well nigh lost, but that DRY, FORMAL, ORTHODOX MEN BEGAN TO RIDICULE WHATEVER THEY HAD NOT THEMSELVES, and to decry them all as either madness or imposture."

Yes, Brother Wesley was lamenting the fact that many of the cold, formal, orthodox men were ridiculing the gift of healing, and in substance they were excusing themselves before their congregations. They had no power with God, they did not fast and pray to have it, therefore, they ridiculed those who did have the divine presence and power of God in their lives. Cold fundamental men who are opposing and ridiculing the gifts of the Holy Spirit will attack what they do not have to excuse themselves before their congregations.

Here is a testimony of a deacon's wife who fasted and prayed. God instantly and miraculously healed her.

HEALED OF A CHILDHOOD AFFLICTION

Feb. 14, 1947
Tacoma (3), Wash.

I wish to give my personal testimony of how the Lord so wonderfully and instantly healed my body.

I tried going on a fast for a few meals, but really *did not understand how to fast for any length of time* until I secured Brother Hall's book on fasting, and read it. I went on an eight-day fast and truly I can say that the Lord has wonderfully HEALED MY BODY. I have had an ailment in my body since early childhood and I also had female trouble. I was completely healed of both of these ailments. Glory to Jesus!

The fast also brought me much closer to the Lord.

I am a deacon's wife and a member of a prominent church in Tacoma, Washington. I regret to say that some folks of our church "shook their heads" at Brother Hall's, Little David's, and Brother Hanson's meetings where hundreds were saved, many healed, and filled with the Spirit. Fasting was objected to mostly, and I was on my fast at this very time. Several of the congregation got healed by fasting and prayer and the pastor's daughter received her baptism at the meeting. Several apologized and took back what they said aganist the FASTING TRUTH.

I am thankful that I got my eyes opened. I have seen greater results in this meeting than any meeting that ever came to the city of Tacoma. There were larger crowds, more healings, more people were saved, and more received the Holy Ghost baptism than in any other meeting that ever came to this city. I can see that fasting and prayer works.

Sincerely,

Mrs. R. R.

Martin Luther also believed and practiced Divine Healing and fasting and prayer. He spent weeks in fasting when translating the Bible. Melancthon was dying and, in answer to Luther's prayer, was healed.

Dr. A. J. Gordon was one of the greatest Baptist teachers and scholars. He was pastor of the famous Clarendon Street Church in Boston, and under his profoundly spiritual ministry, that church experienced a transformation which was nothing short of miraculous. He laid due emphasis upon this truth of Divine Healing as well as upon fasting and prayer.

Charles Spurgeon of London Baptist Tabernacle, prayed for many sick who were healed. Dr. Roach Strat-

ton of the Calvary Baptist Church of New York, prayed
for the sick, and many were healed.

When the Protestant Episcopal Convention met at
Washington, D. C., October 22, 1928, the general convention listened to a report of a joint commission of
bishops and deputies, which declared that: "Christian
healing has passed beyond the state of experiment, and
its value cannot be questioned." This was accepted after
six years of studying the results of Divine Healing. Mr.
Hickson, an outstanding Episcopalian layman toured the
British Empire and America praying for thousands of
Episcopalians and many were healed in answer to prayer
and fasting. Many Episcopalian churches now have regular divine healing services in which the sick are anointed
with oil and prayed for.

If healing for the body was not in the atonement,
why were types of the atonement given in connection with
healing throughout the Old Testament? Why were the
dying Israelites required to look at the type of the Atonement for bodily healing?

The slogan of the ages is "Look and Live," or HEAL-
ING FOR A LOOK, either forward to the Cross, or now
since Christ died and arose, backward to the Cross upon
which Christ died, and away through the balconies of
heaven where He ever liveth to make intercession for us—
yes, for our healings as well as for forgiveness of sins.
Look to the Lamb of God and LIVE, both body and
Spirit. This was why the dying Israelites were required
to look at the type of the Atonement for bodily healing.

SUGAR COATED PILLS WITH THE SUGAR REMOVED

If healing was not provided for all in redemption,
how did the multitudes obtain from Christ that which
God did not provide?

If the body was not included in redemption, how
can corruption put on incorruption, or mortality put on
immortality? Were not the physical as well as the spiritual earnests (samples) of our coming redemption enjoyed by God's people throughout history?

Why should not the second Adam take away all the
curse that the first Adam brought upon us?

If the Church is the body of Christ, is it not logical
to believe Jesus does not want His body sick? Is it not

His will to heal any part of His body, as well as the soul?

Are physical, moral or any other human imperfections God's will, or are they man's mistakes?

How can Christ make us "perfect in every work to do His will" or have us "thoroughly furnished unto every good work?" This can be done by healing the sick and making us well and healthy.

Since bodily healing in the New Testament was called a mercy, and it was mercy and compassion that moved Jesus to heal all who came to Him, is not the promise of God still true? "He is plenteous in mercy unto all that call upon Him."

If, as some teach, God has another method for our healing today, why should God adopt a less successful method for our better dispensation?

Since Christ came to do His Father's will, was not the universal healing of all the sick who came to Him, a revelation of the will of God for our bodies?

Did not Jesus emphatically say He would continue His same works in answer to our prayers while He is with the Father (John 14:) and is not this promise alone a complete answer to all opposers?

Why should the Holy Spirit who healed the sick before His dispensation began, do less after He entered office on the day of Pentecost? Surely the Miracle-worker did not come into office to do away with miracles.

The second book of Luke, known as the ACTS, are THE ACTS OF THE HOLY GHOST. It is the revelation of the way He wants to continue to act through the church.

If Christ came to undo and destroy the works of the devil, does He want the works of Satan to remain in our bodies? Is He happy to have us to suffer with a cancer, ulcer, tumor, blind eyes, or any physical ills? "You are bought with a price, you are not your own." "Know ye not that your bodies are the members of Christ?" (1 Cor. 6:15.)

Does the fact Christ could do no miracle at Nazareth prove anything except the unbelief of the people; or would it be right to conclude, because of the failure of Christ's disciples to cast out the epileptic spirit from the boy, that it was not God's will to deliver him? Christ proved by healing him that it is God's will to heal even those who fail to receive healing. Then He gave to them the full formula to follow, in order to be certain of obtaining that which He had provided, and that formula is PRAYER AND FASTING. This will drive out unbelief and generate super-faith to believe and to secure the blessings of healing.

If sickness is the will of God, every physician would be a law-breaker, every trained nurse would be defying God Almighty, every hospital and health resort would be a house of rebellion instead of a house of mercy. We should destroy them instead of supporting them and continually building new ones.

Jesus Christ never commissioned anybody to PREACH THE GOSPEL WITHOUT COMMANDING THEM TO HEAL THE SICK. How can we obey the full and complete Gospel command if there is not the GOOD NEWS (gospel) of healing to proclaim to the sick as a basis for their faith? How could there be faith if there is no good news for them to hear, since "Faith cometh by hearing." The Gospel of Christ is "the POWER OF GOD UNTO SALVATION." The word "Salvation" implies deliverance, and also means HEALING, SAFETY, SOUNDNESS and PRESERVATION.

Next to the subject of fasting, the author believes divine healing and the gifts of the Spirit are more neglected than any other Gospel truth.

Christ died for the whole man, not part of him. There is health for body, soul, and spirit. The Holy Spirit is the One who quickens. He heals and regenerates and makes us partakers of Christ's Divine nature. The Holy Spirit raised Jesus from the dead and He played a prominent part in creation. The Holy Spirit is immutable. The Holy Spirit will raise the dead on the resurrection morn. If you believe in the power of the Holy Spirit, it is easy to believe in divine healing. Divine healing is only a foretaste of the resurrection life.

MANY SICKNESSES AND DISEASES ARE SIN

Many of God's people who are ill are sick because of certain faults in living and eating. This type of sickness is a sin in itself. Health authorities claim ninety-five percent of the American people, including church members, are auto-intoxicated from food poisoning caused by over-eating. The affliction or sickness they have from this "OVERCHARGED WITH SURFEITING" condition, as Jesus Christ has chosen to call it, is a disgrace to the cause of God. See Psalm 107:17-20.

Medical and health statistics reveal the average individual dies from twenty-five to thirty-five years too soon, because he is more interested in satisfying the HUNGER LUST than he is in prolonging his life. This condition is more deplorable among God's people than appears on the surface. To state these facts more plainly, many are committing a slow form of SUICIDE by the over-use of food, and the failure to FAST to keep the cells cleaned up, but they do not know it. Fasting cleans up the tabernacle of the Holy Spirit, and gives Him a clean place in which to dwell. But the failure to fast and to live an abstemious life for the glory of Christ has PREVENTED MANY SICK CHRISTIANS FROM RECEIVED ADDITIONAL HEALINGS.

Facts are facts. God in His love and mercy is a great economist, and the plain teaching of His unadulterated Word makes clear it is not His plan to undo, in a contradictory manner, any law He has given to man for his well being. He will not continually heal sick people and allow them to go out and gorge themselves sick again. It is sin to eat until one gets sick, life itself is shortened, and it is also sinful to tempt God to heal one in order that he MAY CONTINUE TO STUFF AND CRAM UNTIL THE VERY PRESENCE OF GOD IS STUFFED OUT OF HIS LIFE.

Please study Psalm 78; 107:17-20, Deuteronomy 28, Matthew 6, and many other scriptures along these lines. III John 1:2: "Beloved, I wish above all things that thou mayest prosper and be in health, even as thy soul prospereth." Spiritual welfare and prosperity is a first essential, before one seeks the natural food. If one puts God first, he will not be interested in taking so much food, it will ruin his physical health; consequently his body would glorify God better, and would be free from many of the ills which come from wrong eating. We pamper and please our carnal appetites much more than God intended for us to do. Matt. 6:33: "Seek ye first the kingdom of God and His righteousness; and all these things shall be added unto you." What "THINGS?" The things "your FATHER knoweth ye have need of." (Matt. 6:32) This takes in everything, food, clothing, physical welfare, healings, and every other essential.

Many sinners, when they come to Jesus, can obtain healing more quickly than Christians who have been saved for some time. The reason for this is simple: Christians have had many opportunities to follow Christ's pattern of abstemious living, while the sinner needs an opportunity, and a chance to be shown the way. On the other hand, the Christian sometimes neglects to live right, and his healing would only be an excuse for over-indulgence again.

Our Father is loving and forgiving, and sometimes He heals the body and winks at ignorance of the better and more holy way of living, even though the healings may prove a disadvantage to the spiritual and physical welfare at some future time.

Many times He forgave their misdeeds, and granted certain petitions to the children of Israel when it was not to their best interest, but because they cried unto Him until He answered.

James reveals to us interesting information along this line. James 4:3: "Ye ask, and receive not, because ye ask amiss, that ye may consume it upon your lusts." I believe it is God's will to heal the sick, but if an individual is seeking to be healed so he can eat anything under the sun to satisfy his lustful appetite, I believe the individual is asking amiss. He needs to turn his first attention to the spiritual man, then later he will have a healing with such a spiritual blessing it will be for the Glory of God to the fullest extent. Again we go to James 5:15: "The prayer of faith shall save the sick, and the Lord shall raise him up; and if he have committed sins, they shall be forgiven him." These sins include the sin of overeating.

Since we are dealing with some reasons why people are not healed, I wish to state that many times a Christian is sick or afflicted, not because of intemperate living, or because of sin, but that God may be Glorified, and Jesus exalted.

"Many are the afflictions of the righteous but the Lord delivereth him out of them all." Psalms 34:19. We will have suffering and sickness as long as we remain in this sin-cursed world, but thank God we can be delivered.

"BECAUSE OF YOUR UNBELIEF"
MATT. 17:20
WELLS OF MUDDY WATER
FOOD ABSTENTION RELEASES ENERGIES TO START "HOUSE CLEANING"

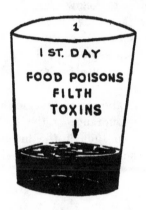

1ST. DAY

FOOD POISONS FILTH TOXINS

FOOD ABSTENTION BEGUN

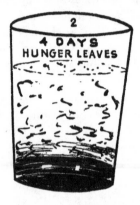

4 DAYS HUNGER LEAVES

THE PROCESS OF OXYGENATION

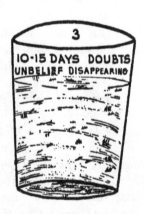

10-15 DAYS DOUBTS UNBELIEF DISAPPEARING

AFTER WEAKNESS THE FAST PROPER

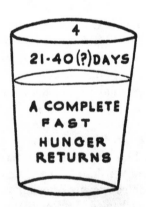

21-40 (?) DAYS

A COMPLETE FAST HUNGER RETURNS

PHYSICAL & SPIRITUAL PURIFICATION

Fasting stirs up physical filth as well as carnality. Both physical impurities and unbelief are eradicated during fasting. Fasting enables us to see unbelief.

The depression, remorse, humility, and great undone feeling into which one will be brought by the fast, plus the great curative cleansing of the body through the automatic blood transfusion and purification, brings one up to the greatest of spiritual heights. However, this is not fully realized and appreciated until after the fast. Fasting is a gruelling process, but Jesus Himself promises every follower a REWARD. Let us more earnestly seek Him through this great medium. It so glorifies Him. It exalts Him because it humbles us, and makes us nothing, and as the result of it all, we do amount to more in His precious sight. Whatever the cost in travail and misery which may be experienced while fasting, the reward is great, and glorious afterward. Taste, try, experience, and see; you will also agree with the thousands of others who are even now in their fourth and fifth major fast of ten days, two weeks, three weeks and even forty days.

While in Portland, Oregon, I organized a FASTING CHAIN through teaching upon the subject of fasting. There was the Wings of Healing Prayer chain. They really knew how to pray but knew little about fasting.

Ninety days later we came back to Portland to the Civic Auditorium which seats 5,000 people. The fasting chain had been in operation and earnest Christians had been fasting for weeks. The results were very gratifying Hundreds were converted, and scores received the Baptism of the Holy Spirit, Hundreds definitely received healing for their bodies and this large auditorium had its first major divine healing service. (See photo)

Although this wonderful healing prayer chain had received many testimonies to healings, before they fasted, after incorporating continuous fasting in to the prayer chain, many more healings resulted.

Our evangelistic group was more than pleased with the results. Little David, twelve-year-old boy preacher, (a product of a 14 day fast), is shown in white in the middle. Doctor Thomas Wyatt is on the right, and next to him is Sister Wyatt. To the left of Little David is the author of this book, Franklin Hall, and to his left, Little David's sister (age 14), who recently concluded a ten-day fast for the salvation of sinners. The next three girls are The Rose of Sharon Trio, the Gering sisters of our party. From right to left, Jo Ann who is on a ten-day

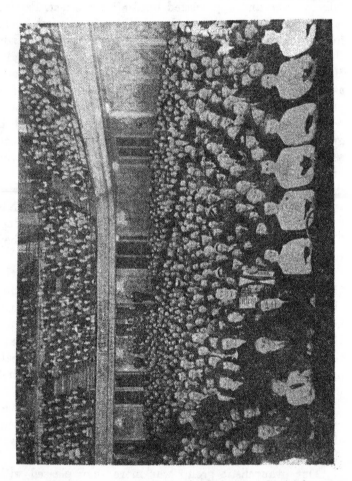

Results of fasting and prayer in Portland, Oregon. Portland municipal auditorium seating 5,000. (Only half of crowd shown.) Ninety days prior to this city campaign, a continuous fasting chain was organized. Hundreds of people began fulfilling Joel 2:12. Approximately four hundred came seeking salvation and scores testified to being healed. Many received the Holy Spirit and His works. Our evangelistic party concluded a ten day fast before this meeting. Little David and Doctor Thomas Wyatt are seated to the right of author in front row. First healing service in this auditorium.

fast, next is Joyce, who is also on a ten-day fast, and
Gladys, who is on her fourteen-day fast. These three
sisters concluded their ten-day fasts and the fourteen-day
fast in Salem, Oregon, where God mightily moved and
hundreds were converted, baptized and healed. See Auditorium picture of Salem elsewhere.

The three Gering sisters testified that they never felt
so fine in their lives.

For further verification of the greater results reported
by a prayer group that took on fasting in a major way,
and included a continuous fasting chain in their midst, the
sister who is at the head of this Prayer group wrote the
following letter to me three months after the continuous
fasting chain was started. Doctor Thomas Wyatt, who
has a "coast to coast" broadcast, is pastor of the "Wings
of Healing Church."

Portland, Oregon
Dec. 2, 1946

Dear Brother Hall:

"Praise God, I came out so victorious
in my twelve-day FAST. It seems I was
pressed into the wilderness to pray — being
under a heavy burden for the HEALING
MINISTRY of which I am in charge and also
for souls in the church. It was as if two angels
came and carried me away to a cabin near the
ocean, and in the mountains to be alone with
God. It seemed as if I was continually in the
presence of the Lord. THESE WERE SOME
OF THE MOST PRECIOUS MOMENTS
OF MY LIFE as I feasted on the good things
of God. I gained spiritual heights I never before have gained, and many prayers were
answered. Spiritual gifts began to be stirred
up.

"May I also state that since our group
has taken on this fasting chain, five times
more testimonies of major definite healings
have been pouring in like a flood. This is a
result of praying and fasting over hundreds of
requests in letters that have come in through
the Wings of Healing Broadcast.

"I recommend very highly the teaching

in the book, 'Atomic Power with God through Fasting and Prayer'.

"Thank Jesus it pays to fast as well as pray."

Sister Peggy Arns,
Wings of Healing,
Box 48
Portland 7, Oregon

The following testimonies came in, in approximately one week, to the Wings of Healing as to results of fasting and prayer. These are only a few of the many healing testimonies. Space will not permit the publishing of them all. We present them here for the Glory of God, in the hope that more faith and power will be developed through the "FASTING PRAYER," by God's SPIRIT.

HEALINGS THRU THE FASTING-CHAIN PRAYER GROUP

Wings of Healing
Portland, Oregon.

Paralysis HEALED

Omaha, Nebraska

My little girl who had been paralyzed is now getting along fine. Since you have been praying for her, she has been MARVELOUSLY HEALED. I just can't keep her still, she is so active. I'm so thankful for your prayers, and praise God for what He has done.

Rheumatism All Over

Winthrop, Ark.

Thank you for praying for me. I have touched the hem of His garment since you prayed for me. I had rheumatism in almost every joint in my body, and suffered so intensely I felt like destroying myself. Friends prescribed many cures but none of them helped, however one day I wrote to your FASTING PRAYER GROUP. After a few days every ache and pain left me immediately. I met the Lord Jesus, and He delivered me from that spirit of infirmity. May God bless you for all of your prayers of faith.

Epilepsy

Atlanta, Iowa

Thank God for answering your sincere prayers and delivering me from epilepsy. I had been bound with this terrible thing for so many years that I was in the very depths of despair. I feel so unworthy because I know I did not deserve help from the Lord, but I know it was because He loved me so much.

Ear Trouble

Mc Clelland, Iowa

For ten years I have been bothered with ear trouble and head noises. After you prayed the prayer of faith for me, Jesus stepped in and healed me completely. I do thank the Lord for this answer to prayer.

Crippled Child

Silverton, Ore.

Our daughter received a wonderful healing through your prayers. She had been afflicted in her feet and legs from birth and as she grew older her lower back and hips were becoming terribly affected. In despair we were about to take her to the hospital for crippled children.

We heard of your healing ministry and brought her to your church where a lot of folk were on a fast and prayer. Our daughter received a wonderful healing through your prayers. She is perfectly normal now, thank Jesus.

Heart Trouble

Tulsa, Okla.

Praise the Lord, "He is the same yesterday, and today, and forever." Our minister has always told us that healing was not for us today. He says these things were just for the days of the apostles but the Lord has proved to me and everyone in our community he still delivers and performs miracles today, the same as He always did.

I have suffered with my heart for many years and had become very nervous and weak as a result of it.

I wrote in and asked for prayer and Jesus answered, and I have been completely made whole. People in this community are surprised how God answered and healed me.

Heart Attacks

Boulder City, Nevada.

The dear Lord healed me of those heart attacks completely in answer to your prayers and fastings. Praise the Lord.

Very Sick

Shelton, Wash.

I was very sick this week and my granddaughter wrote for prayer for me, and God healed me the very next day. I surely thank you for praying.

Ulcer

I wrote to you in regard to prayer for an ulcer. Soon it began drying up, and in two weeks it was all gone. My health was restored. I can not remember when I had been without a bad breath, but now, thank God, my breath is as sweet as a baby's breath.

Cancer

Mrs. A. E. R.
Bradley, So. Dakota

My father went to your church to be ministered to for deliverence from cancer. We are all praising God at this time for the complete healing of father.

Cancer

Stanton, Iowa

I am so thankful to you and your prayer-fasting band for praying for me for cancer. One day shortly after I wrote you, I felt the Healing Power of God flow through my entire body, penetrating to all the sore places. Now I can truly praise God, for all the soreness is gone, and I am feeling fine, and gaining my strength. How wonderful it is to have my health completely restored once more!

Sinners at Death's Door

Worthington, Mo.

My husband and I have been down to death's door. Jesus completely healed us both. We have both been born again— passed from death unto life. We are both over 50 and thank the Lord for the double work that He has done for us.

Cancer

Jefferson, Iowa

I wrote in asking prayer for my husband who had cancer on the back of his neck. He had doctored it for seven years, but Jesus answered your prayers and completely healed it. Oh, how we glorify the Lord.

Brain Hemorrhage

Portland, Orogon

My husband was not expected to live. The doctor said it was a brain hemorrhage. We called our friends, and the Wings of Healing. Many were on a fast, and after they prayed for him, God raised him up and he WALKED RIGHT OUT OF THE HOSPITAL PERFECTLY WELL.

Digestion Trouble

Arvada, Colo.

I want to thank you for your prayer. The Lord has wonderfully healed my digestive organs in answer to prayer.

Skin Disease

Henderson, Iowa

I am praising the Lord for healing from this terrible skin disease. Praise the Lord for complete victory over sin and disease.

Rheumatism and High Blood Pressure

St. Helens, Oregon

I have been healed of so many things—rheumatism, high blood pressure, and weak eyes. I am so happy to be well again, in answer to your prayers.

Sick Daughter

Portland 1, Oregon

I praise God for answering your prayers and fastings. For four months I have been praying for my sick daughter and she has been under the doctor's care a long time. Now God instantly healed her and she no longer needs the doctor.

Cancer

Woodbine, Iowa

I was anointed, and prayed for for the cancer that I had on the back of my head. Thank Jesus for healing me. I am telling everyone about this great healing. O how wonderful the Lord is to us, and we give Him so little thanks.

Affliction

Oberlin, Kansas

I received the blest handkerchief from your FASTING-PRAYER group. Thank you so much for it. I received a healing touch in my body for which I do praise the Lord. This affliction disappeared entirely, thank the Lord.

Hiccoughs

Last week I sent you a telegram asking that you pray for a friend in the hospital who had hiccoughs for over two weeks continually, day and night. Doctors could not stop them.

The same day that I wired you, the hiccoughs stopped. Praise Jesus, the Great Physician.

Appendicitis

Blue Springs, Neb.

My daughter had a strep throat and was to have an operation for appendicitis. Her fever ran up to 106 and in a dying condition we called you. Immediately her fever broke and the doctors could not understand the sudden change. We know it was the Lord. Our daughter is home from the hospital and feeling perfectly well.

Tuberculosis

North Topeka, Kansas

I want to thank you and the prayer band. My son was completely delivered, by the hand of God, from tuberculosis. The X-rays show the old scars on the lungs are not active. I give God glory.

Ulcers of the Stomach

Red Oak, Iowa

My husband who had ulcers of the stomach is completely healed. He is now feeling fine, working every day and weighs more than he ever did. God healed in a wonderful way.

Tumor

Mrs. A. C. S.
Nebraska City, Neb.

My daughter who was very ill with tumor is now completely well and healed in answer to your prayers. The doctor said that she no longer had the tumor.

Sugar Dibetes

J. B.
Portland 6, Ore.

I thank Jesus for completely healing me of sugar diabetes, with which I suffered for so long.

Anemia and Heart Trouble

Mrs. A. D.
Center, Mo.

I was going to the doctors once a week for treatment of my heart trouble and anemia. He informed me that an operation was necessary. I was getting worse and decided to give up the doctor. When I reached my extremity, I wrote in to ask for prayer and thank the good Lord, He reached down and completely healed me. I feel better now than I have felt in a very long time.

Arthritis

Mrs. E. K.
Litchfield, Neb.

Thank God for healing me of arthritis in answer to prayer and the blest hankerchief. My daughter was also healed.

Sore Leg and Hurting in Breast

Grants, N. M.

Oh, how happy I am that my husband has been healed by your prayers. My husband had a sore on his leg that he has had over a year. Praise the Lord for completely healing him. Jesus also healed my breast that was severely hurting me. I know He answers prayers.

High Blood Pressure and Heart Trouble

Portland, Oregon

I was sick all the time with heart trouble, high blood pressure, and stomach trouble. I was in such pain that I did not want to live. After my daughter called up your FASTING PRAYER BAND, the Lord delivered me immediately. We had a real time of praise and thanksgiving afterward.

Cancer

Livingston, Mont.

I thank you from the bottom of my heart for the blest hankerchief that we received from your fasting-prayer chain. We placed it upon my husband's body in the name of Jesus. He was not instantly healed, but he is well on the way to recovery. The doctor had given him up to die with cancer, so we are so thankful to the Lord for what He is doing.

Healed of Gall Stones, Cancer of the Liver and Sinus Trouble

On February 17, 1946, I had an attack of gall stones; I suffered the most intense pains in my right side. On Feb. 19, 1946, I was suffering so terribly that I had a doctor. He said I had gall stones and cancer of the liver in the last stage. It would be a miracle if I lived, he told me. I was rushed to a hospital and expected to die in a week. They took X-rays and doctored me but I grew worse.

At the Broadway Revival Auditorium, where I attended church, Bro. Franklin Hall had organized a fasting chain.

Some were fasting two and three weeks and longer at this time I became ill. I sent for one of the ministers of the auditorium, and requested prayer. Bro. Frank Silva came out to the hospital and prayed for me. God bless his soul, he prayed the prayer of faith, glory to God, and Jesus wonderfully and instantly healed me and lifted me up from my death bed. It was four days after I entered the hospital in this dying condition, Jesus healed me. It was a glorious instantaneous healing.

I am 78 years of age and now do all my own work and feel 50 years younger. Praise the good Lord for ever. Glory Hallelujah!

                                    Mrs. M. S. Painter
                                    San Diego, Calif.

Many more fasting healing testimonies are available but the few which have been included here should be sufficient to convince any doubter fasting and prayer is very effective in stirring up spiritual gifts and contacting the *Great Physician.*

Why not organize a continuous fasting chain in your church? It shouldn't be too difficult to do and the gifts would soon begin to operate.

Now if you are a backslider or a sinner, you cannot enjoy this fasting experience like Christ's people can, neither can you have hundreds of other blessings that are for those who know the blessed Lamb of God. If a backslider, I recommend FASTING AND PRAYER as a method to bring you quickly into restoration and favor with God. David chose this method, "I humbled my soul with fasting and my prayer returned unto my bosom." If you are a sinner, and never have been converted, make haste and REPENT before it is too late. "HOW SHALL WE ESCAPE IF WE NEGLECT SO GREAT SALVATION?" Someone says, "I am not worrying because God is too just to send a person to hell." I wish to state if one had an opportunity to appear in Heaven or Hell in his unsaved condition, he would prefer Hell to Heaven because it would be a greater hell for him to be in Heaven face to face with a righteous God, in his unclean and miserable condition, than to go to Hell. So God, in His goodness, is righteous to permit one to go to his own place, a place that would be home to him and his fellows. 1 Peter 4:18: "If the righteous scarcely be saved, where shall the ungodly and the sinner appear?" Even the very righteous have difficulty standing up under the holy presence of Christ. Rev. 1:17: "When I saw him, I fell at His feet as dead." John was a holy man, and fell down as dead when he saw Jesus in His glory. Where could an ungodly unsaved sinner appear? I personally believe John was in fasting at this time, because in other instances in the Scriptures when holy men came in contact with God in that way, they were on a fast. Fasting will bring one further into the spiritual realm and nearer to God than any other process known, therefore, it is logical to believe John had been fasting on the Isle of Patmos. Visions such as he saw, are usually a product of fasting.

Let us go to another prophetic book, and see another righteous man who saw a vision similar to the one John saw. Daniel had been on a fast for "three whole weeks". In all of his righteousness, he also fell down as dead when he saw Jesus in His Glory. See Daniel 10:2-9.

To enjoy eternal life, and to be able to go to the place where Christ's own redeemed are, one has to be born into Christ's Kingdom. All sinners must be born again.

A sinner's girl friend whom he loved very much, married another boy. He was so grieved over the jolt, he was going to commit suicide. He did not wish to shoot himself because that would be bloody, he did not want to take poison because that would look cowardly. He decided to starve himself to death, and commit suicide in that manner. Seventy days went by without his eating any food, and he still found himself alive. He felt God did not want him to die. He had plenty of time to think things over and someone also prayed for him. An overruling, supernatural power kept speaking and dealing with him, he gave his heart to the Lord after fasting for seventy days.

May you find the prophecies in the first and second chapters of Joel fulfilled in your life through fastings today.

If you have a fasting experience, won't you kindly mail it in to me and give permission to publish it?

To have the early church's experience, do as they did. Take a prophet's-length fast.